# Algae - Science and Applications

*Edited by Ihana Aguiar Severo*

Published in London, United Kingdom

Algae - Science and Applications
http://dx.doi.org/10.5772/intechopen.1005951
Edited by Ihana Aguiar Severo

Contributors
Ahmed Aidan Al-Hussieny, Ashraf Goda, Bidyut Baran Saha, Edwin H.W. Leung, Ehab El-Haroun, Einar Ringø, Md. Mushfiqur Rahman, Mir Shariful Islam, Mohamed Ashour, Rafid Fayyaz, Sherine Ahmed, Vahid Morshedi, Zaki Sharawy



First published in London, United Kingdom, 2025 by IntechOpen
IntechOpen is the global imprint of INTECHOPEN LIMITED, registered in England and Wales, registration number: 11086078, 167-169 Great Portland Street, London, W1W 5PF, United Kingdom

For EU product safety concerns: IN TECH d.o.o., Prolaz Marije Krucifikse Kozulić 3, 51000 Rijeka, Croatia, info@intechopen.com or visit our website at intechopen.com.

British Library Cataloguing-in-Publication Data
A catalogue record for this book is available from the British Library

Algae - Science and Applications
Edited by Ihana Aguiar Severo
p. cm.
Print ISBN 978-1-83634-548-0
Online ISBN 978-1-83634-547-3
eBook (PDF) ISBN 978-1-83634-549-7

# Meet the editor

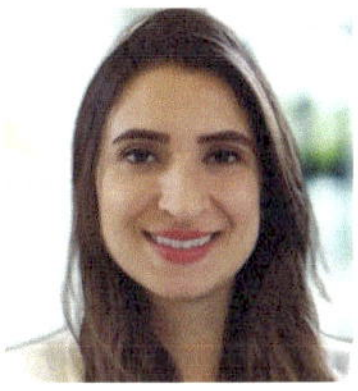

Dr. Ihana Aguiar Severo is a researcher at the Center for Advanced Power Systems (CAPS), Florida State University, USA. She also collaborates as a researcher at the Sustainable Energy Research and Development Center (NPDEAS), Federal University of Paraná, Brazil. She holds a Ph.D. and a master's degree in food science and technology (Federal University of Santa Maria, Brazil). In addition, Dr. Severo has experience in food science and technology with a focus on microalgal biotechnology. Her scientific and technological research interests include microalgae-based processes and products, photobioreactors, process integration, renewable energy, and environmental sustainability.

# Contents

# Preface

Algae have long been recognized as organisms of significant scientific and commercial interest, offering diverse opportunities for sustainable applications in various industries. These remarkable organisms, ranging from microscopic phytoplankton to giant kelp, are more than just the base of aquatic food chains, they are proving to be valuable allies in addressing a host of global challenges.

This edited volume, entitled *Algae – Science and Applications*, presents a comprehensive exploration of algae's multifaceted roles and applications, providing readers with an accessible overview of current developments and uses of algae in various sectors. The book demonstrates how algal science translates into practical solutions in commerce, environmental sustainability, health, and nutrition.

The book explores the commercial and industrial uses of algae, highlighting their growing role in producing biofuels, biodegradable plastics, pigments, and nutritional supplements. Improvements in large-scale cultivation have increased the economic viability of these sustainable applications. The discussion then moves to macroalgae, or seaweeds, highlighting their significant contributions to aquaculture through improved water quality, reduced environmental impact, and diversified farming practices. Next, the environmental benefits of algae are presented through microalgae grown in photobioreactors designed to capture carbon dioxide emissions and convert them into valuable biomass. In addition, algae's pharmaceutical potential is explored, highlighting their rich array of bioactive compounds useful for antimicrobial, anti-inflammatory, and anticancer applications.

Finally, the role of algae as sustainable feed additives in aquaculture is presented, highlighting their nutritional and immune-enhancing benefits for farmed aquatic animals.

The editor would like to thank all the authors for their contributions and knowledge.

**Ihana Aguiar Severo**
Sustainable Energy Research & Development Center (NPDEAS),
Federal University of Paraná (UFPR),
Curitiba, PR, Brazil

Department of Mechanical Engineering,
FAMU-FSU College of Engineering,
Center for Advanced Power Systems (CAPS),
Florida A&M University, Florida State University,
Tallahassee, FL, United States

Chapter 1

# Commercial and Industrial Algae Culture and Applications

*Mir Shariful Islam, Bidyut Baran Saha,*
*Md. Mushfiqur Rahman and Rafid Fayyaz*

## Abstract

Algae, photosynthetic organisms ranging from microscopic to macroscopic forms, play a critical role in carbon sequestration, oxygen production, and maintaining aquatic ecosystem balance. Their extensive applications in pharmaceuticals, biofuels, and bioproducts have positioned algae cultivation as a promising solution for sustainable resource production. Both microalgae and macroalgae can be cultivated using open systems (e.g., longline culture, floating nets, bottom culture, raceway ponds, and saline aquaculture) and closed systems (e.g., photobioreactors, tank cultures, and fermenters). While closed systems offer precise control over growth conditions and productivity, open systems are more cost-effective but susceptible to environmental variability and contamination. Integrated multi-trophic aquaculture (IMTA) enhances resource efficiency by combining algae cultivation with other species, supporting environmental and economic sustainability. This chapter provides an in-depth analysis of algae culture techniques, their industrial applications, and associated challenges. Additionally, the chapter examines future research directions and the role of policy frameworks in advancing sustainable algae culture, offering valuable insights for researchers, industry stakeholders, and policymakers.

**Keywords:** algae culture, open system algae culture, closed system algae culture, IMTA, photobioreactors, fermenters, saline aquaculture

## 1. Introduction

Algae are a highly diverse group of photosynthetic organisms with an extensive fossil record, broadly classified into *macroalgae* and *microalgae* [1]. Macroalgae, or seaweeds, are predominantly found in the littoral zone and include green (*Chlorophyta*), brown (*Phaeophyta*), and red (*Rhodophyta*) algae [2], while microalgae are distributed across benthic and littoral zones and dominate the phytoplankton in open oceans. Globally, there are approximately 900 species of green algae, 4000 species of red algae, and 1500 species of brown algae, with about 250 species being commercially significant for applications, such as food production and phycocolloid extraction [3]. Both macroalgae and microalgae represent significant dietary resources due to their considerable concentrations of vitamins, minerals, proteins, and dietary fibers. Algae are particularly rich in a diverse array of vitamins, including β-carotene, which serves as a precursor to vitamin A, several B vitamins (notably B12), and vitamins C, D, E, and K [4]. Additionally, the elevated enzyme activity in algae enhances the bioavailability and digestion of these essential nutrients. Standard nutritional assessments have consistently revealed high carbohydrate content in algae, in addition to a variety of minerals, vitamins, and trace elements such as iodine, further underscoring their nutritional value [5].

Microalgae play a significant role in the food chain and contribute to the production of valuable bioactive compounds across various sectors, such as skincare, pharmaceuticals, and aquaculture [6]. They are highly efficient in removing nutrients and decontaminating heavy metals from wastewater via biofiltration, owing to their superior nutrient absorption capabilities compared to terrestrial plants [7]. Microalgae-based systems offer an environmentally sustainable alternative to conventional wastewater treatment methods, as they do not produce additional pollution and enable biomass reuse [7]. These systems effectively reduce excess nutrients from aquaculture effluent, promoting environmental sustainability. Their high oil content and rapid biomass production make them a promising source for biofuel production [8]. With a nutritional profile rich in amino acids, fatty acids, phytonutrients, and phycobiliproteins, microalgae are free from toxins, making them suitable for both animal feed and human consumption [9]. In aquaculture, microalgae serve as live feed for zooplankton and various growth stages of bivalve mollusks (e.g., oysters, scallops), abalone, crustaceans, and fish, improving growth, protein deposition, disease resistance, digestibility, and carcass quality, while also reducing nitrogen output [10]. The physiological benefits of microalgae, including enhanced stress tolerance and starvation resistance, have led to their growing use as additives in aquaculture, positioning them as a sustainable and multifunctional resource [11]. Macroalgae are rich in bioactive compounds, such as polysaccharides, proteins, polyunsaturated fatty acids, pigments, polyphenols, minerals, and hormones [12]. Recent research highlights their therapeutic potential, with extracts exhibiting antioxidant, anticancer, antiproliferative, and antibacterial properties [13]. These bioactive compounds contribute to the beneficial biological effects of macroalgae, especially in treating cardiovascular disorders like atherosclerosis, hyperlipidemia, hypertension, and thyroid diseases [14]. Polyphenols and flavonoids in algae are particularly noted for their antibacterial and antioxidant properties, with antimicrobial effects linked to compounds like phenols, fatty acids, terpenes, and indoles [15]. The bioactive composition of algae varies among species and is influenced by environmental and geographical conditions [15].

Algae play a vital role in sustaining marine ecosystems while offering significant nutritional and therapeutic benefits. They contribute to reducing carbon dioxide ($CO_2$) emissions through carbon fixation and act as primary producers in marine environments [16]. The increasing levels of $CO_2$ emissions have accelerated climate change, resulting in severe consequences such as cyclones, floods, droughts, rising sea levels, and other environmental threats that endanger humanity [16]. Despite these challenges, global efforts to reduce carbon emissions remain limited or ineffective in many regions [17]. Consequently, developing effective methods to mitigate CO2 emissions and accumulation has become essential. Biological $CO_2$ fixation is considered the most cost-effective and environmentally sustainable solution for addressing this issue [18]. Algae and cyanobacteria demonstrate growth rates far exceeding those of terrestrial plants, with $CO_2$ fixation efficiencies 10–50 times higher [19]. As some of the fastest-growing photosynthetic organisms on Earth, algae exhibit remarkable biodiversity and are responsible for approximately 50% of the global carbon fixation, highlighting their critical role in combating climate change [20]. Algae culture is gaining significant attention due to its therapeutic and nutritional benefits. It is considered a vital component of the blue economy in various countries worldwide. While substantial progress has been made in commercial and industrial algae cultivation techniques, various challenges remain, influenced by species-specific and regional factors. This chapter explores key commercial and industrial algae culture methods, their applications, and the challenges faced, aiming to provide insights into the development and potential of this expanding industry.

## 2. Algae culture techniques

Algae culture, or algae farming, involves cultivating algae for commercial purposes under controlled conditions in onshore facilities, open waters, or coastal regions. Key factors influencing cultivation include nutrient availability, cost of production, product quality, environmental conditions, technology requirements, and initial investments. There are mainly three types of culture techniques, which are commonly used for commercial and industrial algae culture. They are given below:

1. Closed system culture technique

2. Open system culture technique

3. Integrated multi-trophic aquaculture (IMTA) system

### 2.1 Closed system culture technique

Closed systems for algae cultivation offer higher photosynthetic efficiency, improved biomass productivity, and sustainable yields through precise control of environmental conditions while minimizing water loss [21]. Advanced photobioreactors (PBRs), constructed from transparent materials, optimize light utilization and environmental regulation, though their design remains complex. Fermenter-based and tank systems further integrate technologies for precise control of temperature, light, and aeration, ensuring stable and efficient cultivation. Despite higher resource requirements and costs, closed systems are increasingly favored for high-value algae production due to their reliability and productivity [22]. Although primarily utilized for microalgae, these systems can also be adapted for macroalgae cultivation, enhancing sustainable production practices.

#### *2.1.1 Algae culture using photobioreactor*

Phototrophic microorganisms, including algae, cyanobacteria, and photosynthetic bacteria, are cultivated in photobioreactors (PBRs)—specialized systems designed to harness light for photosynthesis [23]. PBRs consist of transparent culture vessels, nutrient supply systems, gas exchange mechanisms (for $CO_2$ input and $O_2$ removal), mixing systems, temperature regulation, and monitoring tools [24]. Various types of photobioreactors are utilized for algae culture, each offering distinct advantages depending on the specific requirements of the cultivation process. For example, microfluidic photobioreactors enable detailed observation of algae cells, either as isolated entities or within clusters comprising multiple species [25]. Shaken photobioreactors, such as orbital shaker flasks, are commonly employed in illuminated chambers with regulated parameters like humidity, pH, temperature, and $CO_2$ [26]. Vertical column photobioreactors, constructed from materials such as polyvinyl chloride (PVC), glass, or plexiglass, are designed to ensure effective light penetration for optimal algal growth. Bubble column photobioreactors, characterized by their cylindrical structure, offer advantages, such as simplicity, low energy requirements, uniform culture conditions, and reduced photoinhibition, making them efficient and easy to operate [27, 28]. Airlift photobioreactors, featuring interconnected cylindrical zones, promote efficient mixing and mass transfer [29]. Flat-plate photobioreactors are favored for their scalability, high surface area-to-volume ratio, reduced oxygen accumulation, and ease of cleaning and maintenance [30]. Stirred-tank photobioreactors, comprising a vessel, agitator, aerator rod, and pump, ensure enhanced biomass production and improved heat, mass, and light transfer [31]. Horizontal tubular photobioreactors, made from transparent PVC or bio-polypropene sheets, maximize light utilization and homogenize cultures through air pump systems [31]. V-shaped photobioreactors utilize light-trapping geometries to enhance photosynthetic efficiency [32]. PBRs are widely used for carbon sequestration, biofuel production, wastewater treatment, and the production of pharmaceuticals and nutraceuticals. They convert algae into renewable biofuels (biodiesel, bioethanol, and biogas) and purify wastewater by removing nutrients and heavy metals. Additionally, PBRs produce high-value compounds such as vitamins, antioxidants, and pigments for human health. By capturing industrial $CO_2$ emissions, PBRs reduce greenhouse gases (GHGs) while generating protein-rich biomass for use in animal feed or human nutrition [33]. *Chlorella vulgaris, Spirulina platensis, Haematococcus pluvialis, Nannochloropsis oculate, Tetraselmis suecica, Dunaliella salina, Phaeodactylum tricornutum, Isocrysis galbana, Secenedesmus obliquus*, *Pyropia* spp., *Rhodomonas* spp., etc., are suitable algae species for culture using photobioreactors [34].

### *2.1.2 Algae culture in a closed tank system*

Algae farming in tanks, especially for experimental and high-intensity cultivation, began in the 1960s in Canada and the USA, with Chile later adopting similar practices. This approach is now widespread in countries, such as the United States, Canada, Chile, Israel, Mexico, Germany, China, and Japan [35]. Tank culture is known for achieving the highest biomass yields per square meter of water surface when compared to other methods. Algae are grown in tanks for various purposes, including waste treatment from farmed animals, production of plantlets for future cultivation, extraction of valuable compounds like agarose and prostaglandins for medical applications, and as food for abalone mollusks (*Haliotis*) [36]. Macroalgae are typically cultivated in large concrete tanks, often with volumes in the tens of cubic meters, to generate significant biomass, though smaller tanks or aquaria are used for research. While tank cultivation offers high yields, it requires considerable energy and expensive equipment, making it less suitable for large-scale commercial use. Algae culture involves developing specific techniques for each species, optimizing conditions such as light intensity, temperature, and nutrient levels. Light exposure is controlled using filters, screens, and additional lighting, while factors, such as tank depth, algae density, and rotational movement, are managed to promote growth. Rotation is induced by injecting compressed air to create water flow. Temperature control is achieved through water circulation systems or by regulating air temperature. Fertilizers are applied based on water exchange schedules, and $CO_2$ and $HCO^{3-}$ are supplied, when necessary. Salinity is managed with fresh water, distilled water, or sea salt, and microbial growth is controlled using bacterial inhibitors. Excess biomass is regularly harvested to maintain optimal productivity. The yield of algae in tanks varies depending on the species and methods used. For example, *Gracilaria tikvahiae* cultivated in small tanks (55 L) with aeration, regular fertilization, high water turnover, and frequent removal of excess biomass can yield between 12 and 40 g FWT $day^{-1}$ (127 t FWT $ha^{-1}$ $year^{-1}$) [37]. Larger tanks (24,000 L) yield similar amounts for *Gracilaria* sp., and *Porphyra* sp. plantlets can produce up to 120 metric tons of fresh weight per hectare over 4 months of cultivation. Spray cultivation, an alternative intensive alga farming technique, involves spraying algae with artificial seawater enriched with mineral salts [38]. This method is more cost-effective than submerged cultivation and offers advantages, such as reduced epiphytism and the absence of algal pests. *Gracilaria chilensis* cultivated under seawater spray can yield between 1.8 and 16 metric tons of dry weight per hectare per year. In comparison, *Ascophyllum nodosum* yields 143 metric tons of fresh weight or 22 metric tons of dry weight per hectare annually. Other species commonly cultivated in closed tank systems include *Ulva lactuca*, *Gracilaria* spp., *Nannochloropsis gaditana*, *Tetraselmis chuii*, *Chaetoceros calcitrans*, *Skeletonema costatum*, *Chlorella pyrenoidosa*, *Spirulina maxima*, *Pavlova lutheri*, and *Thalassiosira pseudonana*.

### *2.1.3 Algae culture by fermenter-based system*

Fermenter-based algal culture involves growing algae in controlled bioreactors, typically for heterotrophic growth, where algae rely on organic carbon sources like glucose or glycerol, instead of sunlight. While less common, autotrophic growth in fermenters using light is also possible. This system offers several benefits over open-pond methods, including continuous year-round production and precise control of environmental conditions, such as temperature, pH, oxygen, and nutrient levels. Species like *Chlorella*, *Schizochytrium*, and *Crypthecodinium cohnii* are well suited for heterotrophic culture, producing valuable products like biofuels and nutraceuticals [39]. Fermenters facilitate faster growth and higher yields than photosynthetic systems by offering precise control over critical parameters. Unlike open-pond systems that depend on sunlight, fermenters operate in dark conditions, offering flexibility and making them ideal for large-scale, industrial applications. This approach is particularly effective for producing dense algal biomass and high-value products, such as proteins, biofuels, and omega-3 fatty acids [40]. Several types of fermenters are used, including batch fermenters, which grow algae until nutrient depletion, fed-batch fermenters, which extend growth by adding nutrients, and continuous fermenters, which allow continuous production by removing biomass and adding fresh medium. Stirred-tank fermenters use mechanical stirring, while air-lift fermenters rely on air bubbles for mixing and oxygenation [41]. The key advantage of fermenter-based cultivation is the ability to maintain optimal growth conditions, resulting in higher biomass yields and cell densities compared to open systems. Additionally, fermenters operate in aseptic environments, minimizing contamination risks. Their scalability makes them suitable for industrial-scale production of high-value chemicals [41]. Algal species like *Schizochytrium* spp., *Crypthecodinium cohnii*, *Chlorella protothecoides*, *Aurantiochytrium limacinum*, and *Euglena gracilis* are commonly cultured in fermenters [42].

## 2.2 Open system culture technique

Open system algae culture involves cultivating algae in natural or seminatural environments, such as offshore or coastal waters, primarily for macroalgae production. By utilizing natural resources like sunlight, water flow, and nutrients, this method minimizes operational costs and infrastructure requirements, making it ideal for large-scale cultivation. Open systems support sustainable aquaculture by enhancing biodiversity, improving water quality, and contributing to carbon sequestration. Additionally, they provide a renewable biomass source for industries such as food, cosmetics, pharmaceuticals, and biofuels, promoting sustainable resource management.

### *2.2.1 Algae culture by raceway pond*

In recent years, the focus of algal research has shifted toward developing large-scale cultivation systems to meet the growing demand for nutraceuticals and biofuels. Among these systems, raceway ponds (RWPs) are widely used due to their affordability and operational simplicity. These shallow, open systems are designed to maximize light penetration, which is critical for photosynthesis. However, their shallow depth poses limitations, such as reduced productivity per unit area and the need for substantial land to scale up operations. A key challenge in RWPs is the inefficient transfer of carbon dioxide ($CO_2$). The shallow design reduces the interaction time between gas and liquid, leading to poor $CO_2$ mass transfer efficiency. Studies suggest that 80–90% of the $CO_2$ supplied to RWPs escapes into the atmosphere, with fixation efficiencies in open systems typically ranging between 10 and 30% [43]. This inefficiency significantly impacts overall system performance. Several factors influence algal productivity in RWPs, including site selection, pond depth, oxygen levels, salinity, light intensity, algal predators, and $CO_2$ availability. Selecting a site with optimal environmental conditions is critical [44], while pond depth must ensure efficient oxygen circulation and nutrient mixing [45]. Adequate light intensity [46] and effective $CO_2$ management are essential to sustain photosynthesis [47], and mechanical mixing systems are required to distribute nutrients, circulate oxygen, and remove excess $CO_2$ and waste materials [48]. Controlling salinity is crucial for preventing algal diseases and ensuring optimal growth [49], while predator management minimizes losses caused by harmful organisms. The effectiveness of RWPs also depends on their design, with factors such as light penetration, nutrient distribution, gas-liquid mass transfer, and bubble retention time requiring careful optimization. Advanced RWP designs, including paddlewheel-driven ponds [50], sump-assisted raceways [51], hybrid systems [52], and manually mixed configurations, address these challenges. Several algal species are well suited for cultivation in RWPs, including *Chlorella* sp., *Scenedesmus* sp., *Haematococcus* sp., *Dunaliella* sp., *Nannochloropsis* sp., and *Botryococcus* sp. [53]. These species are highly adaptable and hold significant potential for applications in the food, feed, pharmaceutical, and biofuel sectors.

### *2.2.2 Algae culture by longline method*

The longline algae culture method starts with careful site selection, ensuring the optimal environmental conditions such as salinity, temperature, and nutrient levels, typically found in protected coastal regions with high water exchange. This approach is primarily applied to macroalgae culture rather than microalgae. Following site selection, obtaining necessary permits from local authorities is crucial for compliance with environmental and maritime regulations. The longline system consists of a main line, made of durable materials like nylon or polypropylene, anchored at both ends and buoyantly positioned at intervals to maintain the correct depth and tension. Seedlings, selected for their rapid growth and compatibility with local conditions, are attached to the longline using biodegradable clips or strings. These seedlings are evenly spaced to optimize growth, water circulation, and sunlight exposure while being protected from strong currents and waves [54]. Successful cultivation requires regular monitoring and maintenance. Weekly or biweekly inspections are essential to check for damage to the longline, buoys, or anchors, as well as to remove debris, fouling organisms, or competing algae that could affect growth. Once mature, typically after 2–3 months, the algae are harvested and transported to processing facilities. Postharvest care, including washing, drying, and storage in a cool, dry place, is necessary to preserve quality. This results in a sustainable and profitable operation. Species suitable for longline cultivation include *Saccharina latissima* (sugar kelp), *Undaria pinnatifida* (wakame), *Gracilaria* spp., *Macrocystis pyrifera* (giant kelp), *Sargassum* spp., *Laminaria digitata* (oarweed), *Porphyra* spp. (nori), *Eucheuma* spp., *Kappaphycus alvarezii*, and *Alaria esculenta* [55].

#### *2.2.3 Algae culture by floating net method*

The floating net method of algae culture, especially for macroalgae, begins with a comprehensive site assessment to identify favorable environmental conditions, including optimal water currents, minimal wave exposure, and suitable water depth (typically ranging from two to ten meters). After confirming these conditions and securing necessary permits, anchors, typically screw or concrete blocks, are strategically positioned to ensure the stability of the floating net system against tides and currents. Durable materials such as nylon or polyethylene are used for the primary nets, which are connected to the anchors. Buoys are placed at regular intervals around the nets to maintain buoyancy, ensuring proper depth for optimal sunlight exposure while protecting the algae from destructive currents. Seedlings are sourced from specialized nurseries or resilient wild populations, ensuring they are free from pests and diseases. These healthy seedlings are then attached to the nets using biodegradable clips or ties, with spacing designed to promote consistent growth and efficient nutrient absorption. Regular maintenance is vital for system success, involving routine inspections of the nets, buoys, and anchors to ensure structural integrity. Cleaning operations are performed to remove waste, fouling organisms, and competing algae that could hinder growth [54]. Algae, specifically macroalgae typically mature within 2–6 months, depending on species and environmental factors. Harvesting is conducted with care to prevent damage to the nets and remaining algae, and the biomass is quickly transported for processing to preserve quality. The floating net technique provides a sustainable and efficient method for algae farming, supporting the economic and environmental sustainability of marine aquaculture. Technological advancements, skilled workforce training, and ongoing research are essential for optimizing productivity and ensuring the long-term success of this approach [56]. Suitable species for cultivation using the floating net method include *Ulva lactuca* (sea lettuce), *Gracilaria* spp., *Porphyra* spp., *Chlorella* spp., *Undaria pinnatifida* (wakame), *Tetraselmis* spp., *Isochrysis* spp., *Chaetoceros* spp., and *Nannochloropsis* spp. [57].

### 2.2.4 Algae culture by bottom-culture method

The establishment of bottom-culture systems for macroalgae cultivation necessitates a thorough evaluation of environmental parameters, including water depth, substrate stability, and nutrient availability, particularly in shallow coastal regions. Horizontal cultivation employs resilient materials such as nylon or polyethylene for culture lines or ropes, which are anchored using metal stakes or concrete blocks placed strategically to ensure stability. These lines are suspended just beneath the water surface to optimize conditions for algae attachment and growth. Seedlings of algae species are carefully evaluated for their compatibility with local environmental conditions and consumer demand. After undergoing disinfection and sorting, the seedlings are attached to the culture lines or ropes using biodegradable yarn or clips. Appropriate spacing is critical, as it ensures even distribution, adequate access to sunlight, and optimal nutrient availability, which are vital for healthy growth. Regular maintenance and monitoring are essential for successful cultivation. These activities include assessing the health of the algae, removing fouling organisms and undesirable species, and providing nutrient supplements, either organic or inorganic, to reduce competition for resources. Environmental monitoring is equally important to identify and mitigate potential negative impacts on local biodiversity and water quality. Harvesting is typically performed by cutting algae from the culture lines or ropes using specialized tools such as knives or shears. Postharvest management plays a crucial role in maintaining quality. This includes promptly cleaning the algae to remove dirt and harmful microorganisms, followed by proper storage in a cool, dry environment to ensure freshness and preserve quality [58]. Macroalgae species suitable for bottom-culture systems include *Gracilaria* spp., *Ulva* spp. (sea lettuce), *Porphyra* spp. (nori), *Sargassum* spp., *Saccharina latissima* (sugar kelp), *Laminaria digitata* (oarweed), *Chondrus crispus* (Irish moss), *Codium fragile* (green sea finger), and *Macrocystis pyrifera* (giant kelp) [59].

### 2.2.5 Algae cultivation by saline aquaculture system

In recent years, saline aquaculture system is a land-based approach that utilizes saline groundwater, which can be sourced from aquifers, temporary or permanent saline lakes, or as a byproduct of coal seam gas extraction. Common cultivation methods include raceways, tanks (with or without recirculation systems), and ponds lined with plastic or compacted soil. A key advantage of saline aquaculture is its ability to repurpose existing agricultural land with access to saline water, reducing the need for additional resources. Additionally, cultivating marine algae in island saline water (ISW) offers a cost-effective alternative to traditional sea farming, providing raw materials for the seaweed aquaculture industry and creating supplemental income with lower financial investment than sea-based farming systems [60]. Research has also shown that cultivating diverse seaweed assemblages can improve nutrient absorption efficiency compared to monocultures. This highlights the need for further exploration into multi-species cultivation systems, which hold promise for enhancing ecological sustainability and productivity. To advance sustainable algae farming, comparing bioeconomic models and increasing public awareness are essential. These efforts can support innovation, drive investment, and promote the widespread adoption of environmentally friendly practices in saline aquaculture [60]. A variety of algae species are well suited for saline aquaculture, including *Tetraselmis* spp., *Isochrysis* spp., *Chaetoceros* spp., *Nannochloropsis* spp., *Ulva* spp., *Gracilaria* spp., *Dunaliella salina*, *Phaeodactylum tricornutum*, and *Thalassiosira pseudonana*. These species are highly adaptable to saline conditions and are valuable for applications in food production, biofuels, pharmaceuticals, and aquaculture industries [61].

## 3. Algae culture by integrated multi-trophic aquaculture (IMTA) technique

Integrated multi-trophic aquaculture (IMTA) is a sustainable aquaculture approach that mitigates environmental issues like eutrophication caused by feed waste and excretion in animal farming. IMTA combines species from different trophic levels, recycling organic and inorganic wastes as resources for others. This interconnected system reduces fertilizer use in macroalgae cultivation while maintaining ecological balance, profitability, and sustainability [62]. In IMTA systems, nutrients such as dissolved ammonia and phosphate from animals like fish, mollusks, and bivalves are absorbed by macroalgae, converting waste into valuable biomass. This process also stabilizes oxygen, pH, and $CO_2$ levels in the water [63]. Research has shown that macroalgae biomass increases when grown near fish farms. IMTA is particularly suitable for species with high summer productivity, fast nitrogen uptake, and strong market value [64]. IMTA contributes to environmental sustainability by improving water, soil, and air quality and supporting carbon sequestration and biofuel production [65]. Macroalgae can replace synthetic fertilizers and pesticides in agriculture, improving soil health while reducing emissions [55]. Feeding algae to livestock has been shown to lower methane emissions. Locally, IMTA reduces eutrophication and enhances marine biodiversity, while globally, it aids in combating climate change through carbon capture. Economically, IMTA provides opportunities for diversification, allowing producers to expand into new markets [66]. Algal products are often highly valued for their environmental benefits, fetching premium prices. With efficient photosynthesis and fast production cycles, macroalgae are a renewable source of bioactive compounds. However, for IMTA to succeed economically, all components must be marketable, either individually or as a collective system. Large-scale IMTA, especially offshore, holds significant potential for carbon mitigation and sustainable resource use. Developing effective farm designs and selecting suitable species can maximize ecological benefits and financial returns, facilitating global adoption of this approach [62]. Macroalgae species well- suited for IMTA include *Ulva lactuca* (sea lettuce), *Gracilaria* spp., *Saccharina latissima* (sugar kelp), *Porphyra* spp. (nori), *Laminaria digitata* (oarweed), *Chondrus crispus* (Irish moss), *Palmaria palmata* (dulse), *Sargassum* spp., *Macrocystis pyrifera* (giant kelp), and *Codium fragile* (green sea fingers). These species not only provide valuable biomass but also play a key role in ensuring IMTA's ecological and economic sustainability.

## 4. Applications of algae

Algae are versatile and sustainable resources with broad applications across industries, including food, biofuels, cosmetics, and pharmaceuticals (**Figure 1**). They are nutrient-rich, serving as sources of alginate and agar, while also being valued for biofuel production, bioremediation, and providing bioactive compounds for pharmaceutical applications [67].

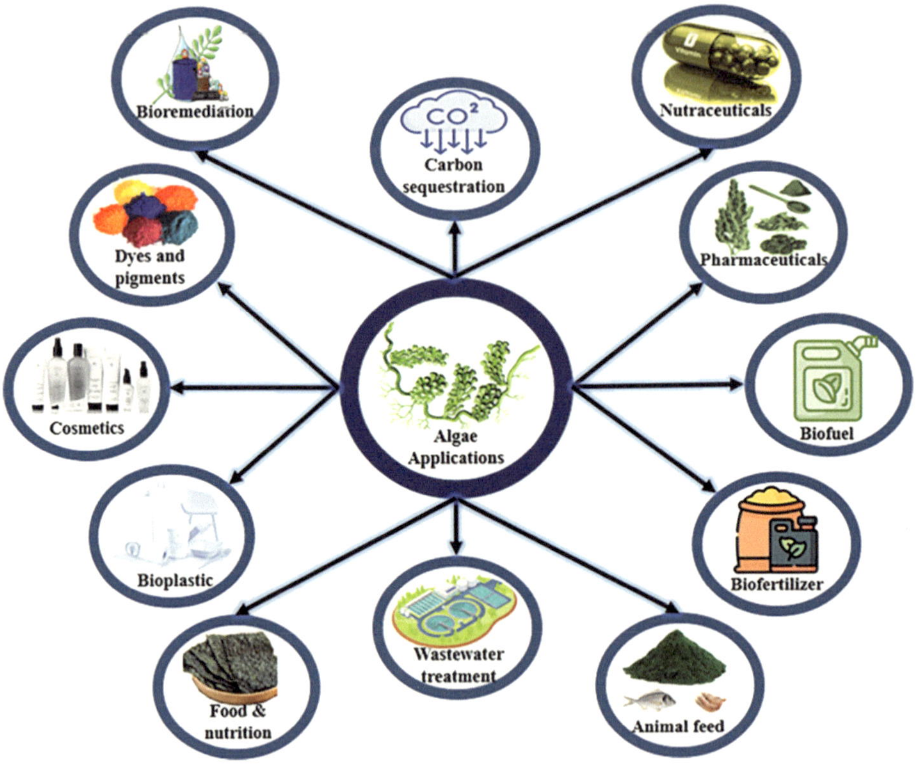


**Figure 1.**
*Diverse applications of algae.*

## 4.1 Food

Micro- and macroalgae have been used as a food source since medieval times in Asia, and with time and increasing awareness of their health benefits in other parts of the world as well [68]. Among the three main components found in any food, proteins, lipids, and carbohydrates, carbohydrate is more common in land-based crops [69]. However, algae contain large amounts of protein and lipids. Moreover, algae contain all the amino acids required for the human diet and are a potential source of omega-3 fatty acids, which are only available through some fish species such as salmon, mullet, and mackerel [69]. These algae are also an excellent source of vitamins and minerals, like potassium and iodine (*Palmaria palmata, Fucus vesiculosus, and Laminaria* sp.), long-chain polysaccharides (*Pyropia tenera*) and dietary fibers (*Grateloupia filicina, Chondrus crispus, and Ulva lactuca*) [70]. Moreover, extracts, such as phycocolloid, carrageenan, and carotenoids, are also used in processed food and are gaining attraction from the industry.

## 4.2 Fuel

With the depletion of fossil fuels and the growing impact of global warming, more research is being done in looking for alternative energy resources. Algal biomass leads to four basic biofuels: biodiesel, bioethanol, biohydrogen, and biobutanol [71]. Due to their high oil-to-dry weight ratio, algae are considered an ideal renewable fuel and energy source, through processes such as transesterification, anaerobic digestion, hydro treatment, fermentation, pyrolysis, and direct combustion [72]. Even though some of these processes are complicated and economically unfeasible, their viability can be achieved through the optimal utilization of all the products.

### 4.3 Cosmetics

Algal biomass is a significant source of biologically active compounds that are scarce in other taxonomic groups [73]. They even have the upper hand over land plants and animal-based foods as they contain a higher concentration of health-promoting elements [74]. These elements are used in foams, humectants, sun protection, soaps, emollients, hair products, shampoos, and lotions [74]. Some of the compounds used in cosmetics that are collected from algae include polyphenols and phlorotannins, polysaccharides, proteins, fucoxanthin, mycosporine, bioactive peptides, and phenolic compounds [73, 74]. These compounds not only help in anti-cellulite procedures and issues such as tanning and pigments disorder, but they also have attributes like antimicrobial, antioxidant, moisturizing, viscosity controlling, whitening, lipolytic, antiphotoaging, and anti-aging [74].

### 4.4 Pharmaceuticals

Polysaccharides are among the most common and active compounds found in algae. These molecules can attach to the surface of leukocytes and reduce inflammation [75]. Fucoidans, sulfated polysaccharides extracted from *Undaria pinnatifida, Laminaria cichorioides,* and *Fucus evanescens* exhibit a wide range of biological activities, including anti-allergic effects, antiviral properties against herpes simplex virus (HSV), respiratory syncytial virus (RSV), and human immunodeficiency virus (HIV), anticancer activity, induction of apoptosis, inhibition of tumor cell growth, and enhancement of chemotherapeutic agents' efficacy [76]. Alginate is another significant polysaccharide that inhibits the release of hyaluronidase and histamine from mast cells, stimulates toll-like receptors, activates cytokine production, and serves as a base material for the base for the production of controlled-release drug products [77]. Additionally, other polysaccharides derived from algae, such as Porphyran, Carrageenans, and Galactans, have demonstrated effectiveness against allergies and different HSV strains as well as inhibit virus amplification during infection [78]. Carotenoids, another group of bioactive molecules extracted from algae, such as fucoxanthin, zeaxanthin, and astaxanthin, have significant application in the pharmaceutical industry. These pigments are used to develop treatments for cancer and cardiovascular disease [79]. Terpenoids, another highly valuable class of compounds, exhibit potent pharmaceutical potential, including anti-HIV-1 activities, antibacterial activity against *Staphylococcus aureus*, and anticancer properties [80].

### 4.5 Bioremediation

Another use of algae is bioremediation, specifically through phycoremediation, a process that utilizes algae to absorb elements such as phosphorus, carbon, and trace metals from wastewater as nutrients [81]. Over the year, many species of algae have been identified that are effective in nutrient removal from wastewater, although their efficiency varies across genera. For instance, *Chlorella kessleri* and *C. protothecoides* grow in municipal wastewater, underscoring their ability to adapt [82]. Additionally, algae can also effectively remove heavy metals from wastewater through accumulation and degrade xenobiotics and crude oil, making them valuable for environmental detoxification [83].

In addition to the aforementioned applications, algae hold significant potential as a sustainable feedstock and an eco-friendly fertilizer for soil enrichment. Algae-based bioplastics represent an innovative solution to reduce microplastic pollution and contribute to environmental preservation. Additionally, the natural pigments present in algae make them a valuable resource for the production of environmentally friendly natural dyes and pigments.

## 5. Benefits of algae culture

Algae cultivation offers significant environmental, economic, and health benefits. One of the significant environmental advantages is its ability to remove nutrients such as nitrogen and phosphorus, which helps in reducing eutrophication and improves overall water quality [84]. Additionally, algae sequester carbon dioxide, mitigating climate change by reducing greenhouse gas concentrations [85]. Furthermore, algae can play a vital role in bioremediation, as they can absorb heavy metals and other pollutants, making them valuable in wastewater treatment and environmental detoxification [86]. From an economic perspective, algae cultivation presents opportunities for sustainable biofuels, such as biodiesel and bioethanol [87]. These renewable energy sources can decrease dependence on fossil fuels while contributing to environmental sustainability. Algae are also rich in bioactive compounds, antioxidants, vitamins, and proteins, making them valuable for several industries, including food, pharmaceuticals, and cosmetics. The growth of the algae industry has the potential to create jobs, thereby contributing to economic development [85].

In terms of health benefits, algae are nutrient-rich and can provide essential fatty acids, proteins, vitamins, and minerals. This makes them valuable as food supplements, as functional foods, or as ingredients in various products. Additionally, they serve as sources of antioxidants and polysaccharides, which can contribute to overall well-being. Algae cultivation offers a wide range of benefits, demonstrating its potential to address global challenges across multiple sectors.

## 6. Challenges of algae culture

Algae cultivation at an industrial scale faces numerous challenges related to ecological, operational, and social factors. A primary concern is the control of fouling algae and epiphytes, which compete with cultivated species for essential resources, such as light, nutrients, and substrate. The presence of invasive species significantly reduces photosynthetic rates and growth, often requiring labor-intensive weeding practices that increase production costs [88]. Another issue is the proliferation of grazing animals, which thrive in mariculture farms where single species are cultivated for extended periods. These grazers feed on seaweed crops, decreasing yields, while efforts to control them, such as using pesticides, can have unintended ecological consequences by harming non-target carnivorous species [89]. Additionally, overgrowth by bivalves such as mussels makes seaweeds too heavy, causing them to detach and decay, further polluting water bodies [90]. The availability and quality of planting stock also present significant barriers. Traditional methods relying on cuttings from cultivated or wild stocks often lead to the degradation of genetic diversity and adaptability over time. This results in reduced resistance to environmental stressors, lower productivity, and eventual declines in harvest yields. While algae cultivation is celebrated for its role in mitigating eutrophication by extracting up to 90% of nitrogen and phosphorus from polluted waters [91], it also poses serious environmental risks. Large-scale monoculture, especially in shallow water lagoons, bays, and estuaries, disrupts benthic ecosystems. Native seaweeds, seagrasses, and other organisms often disappear under seaweed farms due to shading, reduced water movement, and sedimentation [92]. The social implications of large-scale algae farming cannot be overlooked. Farms occupying extensive coastal areas hamper traditional fishing and shipping activities. Addressing these challenges requires a balanced approach that integrates sustainable cultivation practices, ecological restoration, and stakeholder engagement.

## 7. Future prospects of algae culture

The future of algae culture presents a significant opportunity for the sustainable production of biomass and high-value products. As outlined by Buschmann et al. [55], there is a global anticipation that phycologists will rise to the challenges associated with harnessing the potential of seaweed biomass. Emphasizing the need for increased efficiency and economic viability, the focus on microalgae production is vital. Research conducted in Tamil Nadu, India, by Remya and Radhika Rajasree [93] indicates a wealth of studies pertaining to seaweed's distribution, resources, taxonomy, culture, harvesting, and utilization. However, there remains a critical need for intensive investigations into industrial and pharmaceutical applications. Large-scale algae cultivation has great potential for sustainable biomass production and high-value products. However, insufficient data limit commercial trials. Future research should focus on identifying suitable species, optimizing cultivation techniques, and exploring genetic modifications to address challenges, such as the low carbohydrate content in algal biomass [94]. Such modifications can enhance the production of lipids and other target compounds, improve the yield of high-value products, and introduce beneficial traits, such as disease resistance [95]. Techniques like the hybridization of marine macroalgae and advanced genetic engineering strategies hold significant promise for improving the efficiency and economic viability of algal biomass utilization [96]. Immanuel and Sathiadhas [97] noted that many women are actively involved in seaweed collection but they are not fully aware about its demand and value. Given the predominance of women in seaweed collection, targeted efforts should be made to enhance their capacity through education on the market demand and value of seaweeds. Finally, the projected costs for marine algae remain significantly higher than those for terrestrial biomass. Nevertheless, through advancements in yields, scale, and operational efficiencies, algae cultivation could become cost-competitive with terrestrial crops [98].

## 8. Conclusion

The growing demand for algae, valued for their bioactive compounds in nutraceuticals and medicine, threatens wild populations due to limited cultured supply and overexploitation. Developing stable culture systems—closed, open, and IMTA—is essential. Research focuses on optimizing metabolism, improving culture techniques, and selecting fast-growing, resilient species. Despite advancements, challenges remain in ensuring sustainability, profitability, and public acceptance. Sustainable algae culture is vital for driving the global blue economy, promoting economic growth, resource conservation, and environmental sustainability.

## Acknowledgements

The authors acknowledge the use of ChatGPT for grammar editing.

## Author details

Mir Shariful Islam[1*], Bidyut Baran Saha[2], Md. Mushfiqur Rahman[1] and Rafid Fayyaz[1]

1 Department of Oceanography, University of Dhaka, Dhaka, Bangladesh

2 International Institute for Carbon-Neutral Energy Research (WPI-I2CNER), Kyushu University, Japan

*Address all correspondence to: mirsharifuldu77@du.ac.bd

## References

[1] El Gamal AA. Biological importance of marine algae. Saudi Pharmaceutical Journal. 2010;**18**(1):1-25. DOI: 10.1016/j.jsps.2009.12.001

[2] Apaydin G, Aylikci V, Cengiz E, Saydam M, Küp N, Tiraşoğlu E. İstanbul'dan toplanan deniz yosunlarinda EDXRF yöntemi kullanilarak metal konsantrasyon analizi. Turkish Journal of Fisheries and Aquatic Sciences. 2010;**10**(2):215-220. DOI: 10.4194/trjfas.2010.0209

[3] Dawes C. Marine Botany. 1998. Available from: https://books.google.com/books?hl=en&lr=&id=IHGIL7az7p0C&oi=fnd&pg=PA1&dq=Dawes,+1981&ots=qEX3H42ZMA&sig=AfJobVBD_Hmr2sXYNPVnQql72xI [Accessed: June 28, 2024]

[4] MacArtain P, Gill CIR, Brooks M, Campbell R, Rowland IR. Nutritional value of edible seaweeds. Nutrition Reviews. 2007;**65**(12):535-543. DOI: 10.1301/nr.2007.dec.535-543

[5] Morrissey J, Kraan S, Guiry MD, Ryan M. A Guide to Commercially Important Seaweeds on the Irish Coast. 2001. Available from: www.bim.ie [Accessed: June 27, 2024]

[6] Islam MS, Kabir KMA, Tanimoto J, Saha BB. Study on Spirulina platensis growth employing non-linear analysis of biomass kinetic models. Heliyon. 2021;**7**(10):e08185. DOI: 10.1016/j.heliyon.2021.e08185

[7] Shariful IM, Maamoun I, Falyouna O, Belal EB, Eljamal O, Saha BB. Biosorption of arsenic from contaminated water: Composite of algae and Fe-Nano particles. Proceedings of International Exchange and Innovation Conference on Engineering & Sciences. 2021;7:218-223. DOI: 10.5109/4738591

[8] Velichkova K, Sirakov I, Georgiev G. Cultivation of Botryococcus braunii strain in relation of its use for biodiesel production. Journal of BioScience and Biotechnology. 2012;**1969**:157-162. Available from: http://www.researchgate.net/publication/271326530_Cultivation_of_Botryococcus_braunii_strain_in_relation_of_its_use_for_biodiesel_production

[9] Islam MS, Kabir KMA, Islam MS, Saha BB. The perception of consumers towards microalgae as an alternative food resource in Bangladesh: A contingent valuation approach. Evergreen. 2023;**10**(1):1-17. DOI: 10.5109/6781028

[10] Becker EW. Micro-algae as a source of protein. Biotechnology Advances. 2007;**25**(2):207-210. DOI: 10.1016/j.biotechadv.2006.11.002

[11] Fleurence J et al. What are the prospects for using seaweed in human nutrition and for marine animals raised through aquaculture? Trends in Food Science and Technology. 2012;**27**(1):57-61. DOI: 10.1016/j.tifs.2012.03.004

[12] Biswas MH et al. Biological investigations of three marine algae Enteromorpha intestinalis, Rhizoclonium riparium and Ceratophyllum demersum collected from the bay of Bengal. Dhaka University Journal of Pharmaceutical Sciences. 2023;**22**(1):81-87. DOI: 10.3329/dujps.v22i1.67098

[13] Kosanić M, Ranković B, Stanojković T. Biological activities of two macroalgae from Adriatic coast of Montenegro. Saudi Journal of Biological Sciences. 2015;**22**(4):390-397. DOI: 10.1016/J.SJBS.2014.11.004

[14] Kuda T, Nemoto M, Kawahara M, Oshio S, Takahashi H, Kimura B. Induction of the superoxide anion radical scavenging capacity of dried 'funori' Gloiopeltis furcata by lactobacillus plantarum S-SU1 fermentation. Food and Function. 2015;**6**(8):2535-2541. DOI: 10.1039/C5FO00668F

[15] Chandini SK, Ponesakki G, Chandini SK, Ganesan P, Bhaskar N. In vitro antioxidant activities of three selected brown seaweeds of India. ElsevierSK Chandini, P Ganesan, N BhaskarFood Chem. 2008•Elsevier. 2008;**107**(2):707-713. DOI: 10.1016/j.foodchem.2007.08.081

[16] Duarte CM, Losada IJ, Hendriks IE, Mazarrasa I, Marbà N. The role of coastal plant communities for climate change mitigation and adaptation. Nature Climate Change. 2013;**3**(11):961-968. DOI: 10.1038/nclimate1970

[17] Islam MS, Senaha I, Nagamatsu K, Yoda Y, Saha BB. Green algae Caulerpa lentillifera cultivation technique utilising CO2 and its social impacts. International Journal of Innovation and Sustainable Development. 2024;**18**(1/2):146-167. DOI: 10.1504/IJISD.2024.135261

[18] Islam MS, Senaha I, Matiar Rahman M, Yoda Y, Saha BB. Mathematical modelling and statistical optimization of fast cultivation of Agardhiella subulata: Response surface methodology. Energy Nexus. 2022;**7**:100115. DOI: 10.1016/j.nexus.2022.100115

[19] Costa JAV, Linde GA, Atala DIP, Mibielli GM, KruÈger RT. Modelling of growth conditions for cyanobacterium Spirulina platensis in microcosms. World Journal of Microbiology and Biotechnology. 2000;**16**:15-18

[20] Ray S, Abraham J, Jordan N, Lindsay M, Chauhan N. Synthetic, photosynthetic, and chemical strategies to enhance carbon dioxide fixation. C. 15 Mar 2022;**8**(1):18. DOI: 10.3390/c8010018

[21] Khanjani MH, Zahedi S, Mohammadi A. Integrated multitrophic aquaculture (IMTA) as an environmentally friendly system for sustainable aquaculture: Functionality, species, and application of biofloc technology (BFT). Environmental Science and Pollution Research. 2022;**29**(45):67513-67531. DOI: 10.1007/s11356-022-22371-8

[22] Wasanasathian A, Peng CA. Algal photobioreactor for production of lutein and zeaxanthin. In: Bioprocessing for Value-Added Products from Renewable Resources. Elsevier; 2007. pp. 491-505. DOI: 10.1016/B978-044452114-9/50020-7

[23] Islam MS, Hossain T, Islam MS, Saha BB. Dynamical behaviour of single photobioreactor with variable yield coefficient. Heliyon. 2022;**8**(12):e12187. DOI: 10.1016/j.heliyon.2022.e12187

[24] Yuvraj AS, Vidyarthi A, Singh J. Enhancement of Chlorella vulgaris cell density: Shake flask and bench-top photobioreactor studies to identify and control limiting factors. Korean Journal of Chemical Engineering. 2016;**33**(8):2396-2405. DOI: 10.1007/s11814-016-0087-5

[25] Westerwalbesloh C et al. A microfluidic photobioreactor for simultaneous observation and cultivation of single microalgal cells or cell aggregates. PLoS One. 2019;**14**(4):1-13. DOI: 10.1371/journal.pone.0216093

[26] Büchs J. Introduction to advantages and problems of shaken cultures. Biochemical Engineering Journal. 2001;7(2):91-98. DOI: 10.1016/S1369-703X(00)00106-6

[27] Manjrekar ON, Sun Y, He L, Tang YJ, Dudukovic MP. Hydrodynamics and mass transfer coefficients in a bubble column photo-bioreactor. Chemical Engineering Science. 2017;**168**:55-66. DOI: 10.1016/j.ces.2017.04.016

[28] López-Rosales L, García-Camacho F, Sánchez-Mirón A, Contreras-Gómez A, Molina-Grima E. Modeling shear-sensitive dinoflagellate microalgae growth in bubble column photobioreactors. Bioresource Technology. 2017;**245**:250-257. DOI: 10.1016/j.biortech.2017.08.161

[29] Ding N, Li C, Wang T, Guo M, Mohsin A, Zhang S. Evaluation of an enclosed air-lift photobioreactor (ALPBR) for biomass and lipid biosynthesis of microalgal cells grown under fluid-induced shear stress. Biotechnology and Biotechnological Equipment. 2021;**35**(1):139-149. DOI: 10.1080/13102818.2020.1856717

[30] Zhao L, Tang Z, Gu Y, Shan Y, Tang T. Investigate the cross-flow flat-plate photobioreactor for high-density culture of microalgae. Asia-Pacific Journal of Chemical Engineering. 2018;**13**(5):1-11. DOI: 10.1002/apj.2247

[31] Singh RN, Sharma S. Development of suitable photobioreactor for algae production - A review. Renewable and Sustainable Energy Reviews. 2012;**16**(4):2347-2353. DOI: 10.1016/j.rser.2012.01.026

[32] Cho C et al. Study of optical configurations for multiple enhancement of microalgal biomass production. Scientific Reports. 2019;**9**(1):1-11. DOI: 10.1038/s41598-018-38118-w

[33] Islam MS, Rahman MM, Saha BB. Full factorial experimental design for growth of Spirulina Platensis and valuable products enhancement. International Exchange and Innovation Conference on Engineering and Sciences. 2020;**November**:299-304. DOI: 10.5109/4102506

[34] Acién Fernández FG, Fernández Sevilla JM, Molina Grima E. Photobioreactors for the production of microalgae. Reviews in Environmental Science and Biotechnology. 2013;**12**(2):131-151. DOI: 10.1007/s11157-012-9307-6

[35] Titlyanov EA, Titlyanova TV. Seaweed cultivation: Methods and problems. Russian Journal of Marine Biology. 2010;**36**(4):227-242. DOI: 10.1134/S1063074010040012/METRICS

[36] Msuya FE, Neori A. Effect of water aeration and nutrient load level on biomass yield, N uptake and protein content of the seaweed Ulva lactuca cultured in seawater tanks. Journal of Applied Phycology. 2008;**20**(6):1021-1031. DOI: 10.1007/s10811-007-9300-6

[37] Hanisak MD. Recycling the residues from anaerobic digesters as a nutrient source for seaweed growth. Botanica Marina. 1981;**24**(1):57-62. DOI: 10.1515/botm.1981.24.1.57

[38] Israel A, Levy I, Friedlander M. Experimental tank cultivation of Porphyra in Israel. Journal of Applied Phycology. 2006;**18**(3-5):235-240. DOI: 10.1007/s10811-006-9024-z

[39] Javed MU, Mukhtar H, Zieniuk B, Rashid U. Algal-based hollow fiber membrane bioreactors for efficient wastewater treatment: A comprehensive review. Fermentation. 2024;**10**(3):131. DOI: 10.3390/fermentation10030131

[40] Uchida M, Miyoshi T. Introduction. 2013;**47**(1):53-63

[41] Doucha J, Lívanský K. Production of high-density chlorella culture grown in fermenters. Journal of Applied Phycology. 2012;**24**(1):35-43. DOI: 10.1007/s10811-010-9643-2

[42] Sarıtaş S, Duman H, Karav S. Nutritional and functional aspects of fermented algae. International Journal of Food Science and Technology. 2024;**59**(8):5270-5284. DOI: 10.1111/ijfs.17297

[43] Richmond A. Principles for attaining maximal microalgal productivity in photobioreactors: An overview. Asian Pacific Phycology in the 21st Century: Prospects and Challenges. 2004;**i**(Table 1):33-37. DOI: 10.1007/978-94-007-0944-7_5

[44] Bennett MC, Turn SQ, Chan WY. A methodology to assess open pond, phototrophic, algae production potential: A Hawaii case study. Biomass and Bioenergy. 2014;**66**:168-175. DOI: 10.1016/j.biombioe.2014.03.016

[45] Sutherland DL, Turnbull MH, Craggs RJ. Increased pond depth improves algal productivity and nutrient removal in wastewater treatment high rate algal ponds. Water Research. 2014;**53**:271-281. DOI: 10.1016/j.watres.2014.01.025

[46] Kumar K, Sirasale A, Das D. Use of image analysis tool for the development of light distribution pattern inside the photobioreactor for the algal cultivation. Bioresource Technology. 2013;**143**:88-95. DOI: 10.1016/j.biortech.2013.05.117

[47] Ketheesan B, Nirmalakhandan N. Development of a new airlift-driven raceway reactor for algal cultivation. Applied Energy. 2011;**88**(10):3370-3376. DOI: 10.1016/j.apenergy.2010.12.034

[48] Hreiz R, Sialve B, Morchain JÔ, Escudié R, Steyer JP, Guiraud P. Experimental and numerical investigation of hydrodynamics in raceway reactors used for algaculture. Chemical Engineering Journal. 2014;**250**:230-239. DOI: 10.1016/j.cej.2014.03.027

[49] Fon Sing S, Isdepsky A, Borowitzka MA, Lewis DM. Pilot-scale continuous recycling of growth medium for the mass culture of a halotolerant Tetraselmis sp. in raceway ponds under increasing salinity: A novel protocol for commercial microalgal biomass production. Bioresource Technology. 2014;**161**:47-54. DOI: 10.1016/j.biortech.2014.03.010

[50] Chiaramonti D et al. Review of energy balance in raceway ponds for microalgae cultivation: Re-thinking a traditional system is possible. Applied Energy. 2013;**102**:101-111. DOI: 10.1016/j.apenergy.2012.07.040

[51] Mendoza JL et al. Oxygen transfer and evolution in microalgal culture in open raceways. Bioresource Technology. 2013;**137**:188-195. DOI: 10.1016/j.biortech.2013.03.127

[52] Adesanya VO, Cadena E, Scott SA, Smith AG. Life cycle assessment on microalgal biodiesel production using a hybrid cultivation system. Bioresource Technology. 2014;**163**:343-355. DOI: 10.1016/j.biortech.2014.04.051

[53] López-Rosales L, García-Camacho F, Sánchez-Mirón A, Martín Beato E, Chisti Y, Molina Grima E. Pilot-scale bubble column photobioreactor culture of a marine dinoflagellate microalga illuminated with light emission diodes. Bioresource Technology. 2016;**216**:845-855. DOI: 10.1016/j.biortech.2016.06.027

[54] Alam MJ, Fayyaz R, Hasan M, Ahmed MK. Analyzing the potential for Padina gymnospora cultivation in

the coastal waters of St. Martin's Island, Bay of Bengal, Bangladesh: Determining the fluctuations of physicochemical property across seasons and locations. Journal of Biodiversity Conservation and Bioresource Management. 2024;**10**(1): 1-14. DOI: 10.3329/jbcbm.v10i1.74488

[55] Buschmann AH et al. Seaweed production: Overview of the global state of exploitation, farming and emerging research activity. European Journal of Phycology. 2017;**52**(4):391-406. DOI: 10.1080/09670262.2017.1365175

[56] Islam MM, Khan MSK, Hasan J, Mallick D, Hoq ME. Seaweed Hypnea sp. culture in Cox's bazar coast, Bangladesh. Bangladesh Journal of Zoology. 2017;**45**(1):37-46. DOI: 10.3329/bjz.v45i1.34192

[57] Khan ABS, Islam MA, Bosu A, Ullah MR, Haque A, Islam MM, et al. Potentialities of seaweed culture in Kuakata coast of Patuakhali, Bangladesh. Bangladesh Journal of Fisheries Research. 2021;**20**(1-2):35-43

[58] Fax BIO. Culturing algae live material care guide background. Flinn Scientific Inc. 2016;**10583**:1-3

[59] Cai Z, Karunakaran E, Pandhal J. Bottom-up construction and screening of algae-bacteria consortia for pollutant biodegradation. Frontiers in Microbiology. 2024;**15**(February):1-16. DOI: 10.3389/fmicb.2024.1349016

[60] García-Poza S, Leandro A, Cotas C, Cotas J, Marques JC, Pereira L, et al. The evolution road of seaweed aquaculture: Cultivation technologies and the industry 4.0. International Journal of Environmental Research and Public Health. 2020;**17**(18):6528. DOI: 10.3390/ijerph17186528

[61] Vijayaram S, Ringø E, Ghafarifarsani H, Hoseinifar SH, Ahani S, Chou CC. Use of algae in aquaculture: A review. Fishes. 2024;**9**(2):63. DOI: 10.3390/fishes9020063

[62] Knowler D et al. The economics of integrated multi-trophic aquaculture: Where are we now and where do we need to go? Reviews in Aquaculture. 2020;**12**(3):1579-1594. DOI: 10.1111/raq.12399

[63] Zheng Y, Jin R, Zhang X, Wang Q, Wu J. The considerable environmental benefits of seaweed aquaculture in China. Stochastic Environmental Research and Risk Assessment. 2019;**33**(4-6):1203-1221. DOI: 10.1007/s00477-019-01685-z

[64] Troell M, Joyce A, Chopin T, Neori A, Buschmann AH, Fang JG. Ecological engineering in aquaculture - Potential for integrated multi-trophic aquaculture (IMTA) in marine offshore systems. Aquaculture. 2009;**297**(1-4):1-9. DOI: 10.1016/j.aquaculture.2009.09.010

[65] Hossain ABMS, Aishah S. Biodiesel fuel production from algae as renewable energy a. B. M. Sharif Hossain, Aishah Salleh, Amru Nasrulhaq Boyce , Partha chowdhury and Mohd Naqiuddin biotechnology laboratory, Institute of Biological Sciences, Faculty of Science, university o. American Journal of Biochemistry and Biotechnology. 2008;**4**(3):250-254

[66] Mazarrasa I, Olsen YS, Mayol E, Marbà N, Duarte CM. Global unbalance in seaweed production, research effort and biotechnology markets. Biotechnology Advances. 2014;**32**(5):1028-1036. DOI: 10.1016/j.biotechadv.2014.05.002

[67] Patel AK et al. Emerging prospects of macro- and microalgae as prebiotic. Microbial Cell Factories. 2021;**20**(1):1-16. DOI: 10.1186/s12934-021-01601-7

[68] Mendes M et al. Algae as food in Europe: An overview of species diversity and their application. Food. 2022;**11**(13):1871. DOI: 10.3390/foods11131871

[69] Diaz CJ, Douglas KJ, Kang K, Kolarik AL, Malinovski R, Torres-Tiji Y, et al. Developing algae as a sustainable food source. Frontiers in Nutrition. 2023;**9**. DOI: 10.3389/fnut.2022.1029841

[70] Yuan YV, Westcott ND, Hu C, Kitts DD. Mycosporine-like amino acid composition of the edible red alga, Palmaria palmata (dulse) harvested from the west and east coasts of grand Manan Island, New Brunswick. Food Chemistry. 2009;**112**(2):321-328. DOI: 10.1016/j.foodchem.2008.05.066

[71] Mahmood T, Hussain N, Shahbaz A, Mulla SI, Iqbal HMN, Bilal M. Sustainable production of biofuels from the algae-derived biomass. Bioprocess and Biosystems Engineering. 2023;**46**(8):1077-1097. DOI: 10.1007/s00449-022-02796-8

[72] Adeniyi OM, Azimov U, Burluka A. Algae biofuel: Current status and future applications. Renewable and Sustainable Energy Reviews. 2017, 2018;**90**(August):316-335. DOI: 10.1016/j.rser.2018.03.067

[73] Thomas NV, Kim SK. Beneficial effects of marine algal compounds in cosmeceuticals. Marine Drugs. 2013;**11**(1):146-164. DOI: 10.3390/md11010146

[74] Bedoux G, Hardouin K, Burlot AS, Bourgougnon N. Bioactive components from seaweeds. In: Advances in Botanical Research. Elsevier; 2014. pp. 345-378. DOI: 10.1016/B978-0-12-408062-1.00012-3

[75] De Jesus Raposo MF, De Morais AMB, De Morais RMSC. Marine polysaccharides from algae with potential biomedical applications. Marine Drugs. 2015;**13**(5):2967-3028. DOI: 10.3390/md13052967

[76] Zhang YM, Chen H, He CL, Wang Q. Nitrogen starvation induced oxidative stress in an oil-producing green alga Chlorella sorokiniana C3. PLoS One. 2013;**8**(7):1-12. DOI: 10.1371/journal.pone.0069225

[77] Lee KY, Mooney DJ. Alginate: Properties and biomedical applications. Progress in Polymer Science. 2012;**37**(1):106-126. DOI: 10.1016/j.progpolymsci.2011.06.003

[78] Talarico LB, Duarte MER, Zibetti RGM, Noseda MD, Damonte EB. An algal-derived DL-galactan hybrid is an efficient preventing agent for in vitro dengue virus infection. Planta Medica. 2007;**73**(14):1464-1468. DOI: 10.1055/s-2007-990241

[79] Gammone MA, Riccioni G, D'Orazio N. Marine carotenoids against oxidative stress: Effects on human health. Marine Drugs. 2015;**13**(10):6226-6246. DOI: 10.3390/md13106226

[80] Tripathi BN, Kumar D. Prospects and Challenges in Algal Biotechnology2017. DOI: 10.1007/978-981-10-1950-0

[81] Mahapatra DM, Varma VS, Muthusamy S, Rajendran K. Wastewater AlgaetoValue-AddedProducts2018. pp. 365-393. DOI: 10.1007/978-981-10-7431-8_16

[82] Li Y, Zhou W, Hu B, Min M, Chen P, Ruan RR. Integration of algae cultivation as biodiesel production feedstock with municipal wastewater treatment: Strains screening and significance evaluation of environmental factors. Bioresource Technology. 2011;**102**(23):10861-10867. DOI: 10.1016/j.biortech.2011.09.064

[83] Suresh B, Ravishankar GA. Phytoremediation—A novel and promising approach for environmental clean-up. Critical Reviews in Biotechnology. 2004;**24**(2-3):97-124. DOI: 10.1080/07388550490493627

[84] Ullmann J, Grimm D. Algae and their potential for a future bioeconomy, landless food production, and the socio-economic impact of an algae industry. Organic Agriculture. 2021;**11**(2):261-267. DOI: 10.1007/s13165-020-00337-9

[85] Wertz J-L, Perez S. Algae in the Bioeconomy. Boca Raton: CRC Press; 2023. DOI: 10.1201/9781003459309

[86] Camia A et al. Biomass Production, Supply, Uses and Flows in the European Union-JRC Science for Policy Report2018. DOI: 10.2760/181536

[87] Dismukes GC, Carrieri D, Bennette N, Ananyev GM, Posewitz MC. Aquatic phototrophs: Efficient alternatives to land-based crops for biofuels. Current Opinion in Biotechnology. 2008;**19**(3):235-240. DOI: 10.1016/j.copbio.2008.05.007

[88] Buschmann AH, Gómez P. Interaction mechanisms between Gracilaria chilensis (Rhodophyta) and epiphytes. Hydrobiologia. 1993;**260-261**(1):345-351. DOI: 10.1007/BF00049039

[89] Buschmann AH et al. Cultivation of Gigartina skottsbergii (Gigartinales, Rhodophyta): Recent advances and challenges for the future. Journal of Applied Phycology. 2001;**13**(3):255-266

[90] Retamales CA, Buschmann AH. Gracilaria-Mytilus interaction on a commercial algal farm in Chile. Hydrobiologia. 1996;**326-327**:355-359. DOI: 10.1007/BF00047831

[91] Lüning K, Pang S. Mass cultivation of seaweeds: Current practices and approaches. Journal of Applied Phycology. 2003;**15**:115-119

[92] Hurtado AQ, Agbayani RF, Sanares R, De Castro-Mallare MTR. The seasonality and economic feasibility of cultivating Kappaphycus alvarezii in Panagatan cays, Caluya, antique, Philippines. Aquaculture. 2001;**199**(3-4):295-310. DOI: 10.1016/S0044-8486(00)00553-6

[93] Remya RR, Sr R, Radhika Rajasree SR. Biodiversity, distribution and utilization of Brown algae in Tamil Nadu coastline. Alternative dispute resolution Journal. 2015;**October 2016**:1-4

[94] Cozier M. Business highlights: Collaboration: Bigger and beta. Biofuels, Bioprod. Biorefining. 2014;**8**(6):743. DOI: 10.1002/BBB

[95] Gimpel JA, Specht EA, Georgianna DR, Mayfield SP. Advances in microalgae engineering and synthetic biology applications for biofuel production. Current Opinion in Chemical Biology. 2013;**17**(3):489-495. DOI: 10.1016/j.cbpa.2013.03.038

[96] Chisti Y. Constraints to commercialization of algal fuels. Journal of Biotechnology. 2013;**167**(3):201-214. DOI: 10.1016/j.jbiotec.2013.07.020

[97] Immanuel S, Sathiadhas R. Employment potential of fisherwomen in the collection and post harvest operations of seaweeds in India. Seaweed Research and Utilisation. 2004;**26**(1&2):209-215

[98] Warner E, Moriarty K, Lewis J, Milbrandt A, Schwab A. 2015 Bioenergy Market Report. Golden, CO (United States): National Renewable Energy Laboratory (NREL); 2017. DOI: 10.2172/1345716

Chapter 2

# Current and Prospective Pharmaceutical Use of Algal Bioproducts

*Edwin H.W. Leung*

## Abstract

This chapter explores the diverse applications of algal biocompounds in human health, focusing on dietary, cosmetic, and pharmaceutical uses. Algae, ranging from macroscopic kelp to microscopic single-celled organisms (including cyanobacteria), are a rich source of bioactive compounds with potential benefits for human health and well-being. This chapter begins by classifying algae and highlighting their historical use as food. It then delves into the current and prospective applications of algal biocompounds, dividing the discussion into three main sections. The first section examines the dietary uses of algae as food supplements and additives, focusing on their role as sources of macro- and micronutrients, natural colourings, thickeners and prebiotics. The second section explores the external use of algal extracts in cosmetics, discussing their applications in anti-aging, whitening, moisturizing, thickening, photoprotection, antioxidant activity and hair care. Finally, the third section investigates the pharmaceutical potential of algal biocompounds, examining their antimicrobial, anti-inflammatory activities, hypertension management, direct cancer treatment and indirect aids, and diagnostic use. This chapter aims to provide a comprehensive overview of the current state of research and commercial applications of algal biocompounds in human health, highlighting their potential to contribute to sustainable food solutions, enhance cosmetic products, and develop novel pharmaceuticals.

**Keywords:** microalgae, macroalgae, supplement, food, cosmetics, pharmaceuticals, medicine, Chlorella, Spirulina

## 1. Introduction

Algae are predominantly aquatic, simple and eukaryotic (nucleated) plants that range from macroscopic kelp to microscopic single-cellular algae. They belong to the kingdom *Protista*, which can be further divided into seven taxa: *Chlorophyta* (green algae), *Charophyta* (stoneworts), *Euglenophyta* (euglenas), *Chrysophyta* (golden-brown, yellow-green algae and diatoms), *Phaeophyta* (brown algae), *Pyrrophyta* (dinoflagellates), and *Rhodophyta* (red algae) [1]. Despite the taxonomical classification, for the purpose of a more holistic discussion of the "algae" commonly referred to, this chapter will also include the prokaryotic cyanobacteria, that is, the blue-green algae.

In fact, there are a lot of active biocompounds that are present in the blue-green algae, in which the coming sections will explore in detail.

In addition to the above scientific classification into the seven taxa, algae are more commonly classified broadly according to their sizes – complex multicellular macroalgae and smaller unicellular microalgae. Macroalgae like kelp had been found consumed directly to supplement the diets of ancient Peruvians who lived in Pampa along the coast of Peru dating back to 2500 B.C. [2]. Microalgae like *Nostoc* spp., at the other end of the size spectrum, had already been consumed by the Chinese over 2000 years ago as a type of food [3].

These photosynthetic organisms are gaining increasing attention as a sustainable and nutritious food source due to their unique nutritional profile and potential for large-scale cultivation. They are abundant in proteins, vitamins, minerals, antioxidants, etc., making them a crucial component of human diets. The United Nations World Food Conference in 1974 even declared *Spirulina* as the best food for the future, because of their richness in iron and protein and safeness to children [4], on top of their nutritious nature.

Commercialized algal products were first available in the late 1960s and early 1970s. *Spirulina* produced in Lake Texcoco was reported to be the first commercial product for human consumption [5]. *Chlorella*, a green alga commonly seen in the market today, was also reported to be used as a protein supplement on other side of the Pacific in Japan in the 1960s [6]. Numerous other brands of products in the market are available nowadays, and some well-known examples include $\beta$-carotene, astaxanthin and lutein.

Despite the wide variety of algae present in the world and more than 50 years of exploration, to date, not many species of algae have been successfully cultivated for food or other commercial applications. Apart from the *Spirulina* and *Chlorella* we have mentioned, some other species under research and trials are *Haematococcus* spp., *Dunaliella* spp., *Botryococcus* spp., *Phaeodactylum* spp. and *Porphyridium* spp. [7].

Nowadays, with the advancement in biotechnologies in the twentieth century, algal biomass and their bioproducts extend beyond just being food and have been used in a diverse variety of industries. For example, they are being used as feedstock for renewable energy production due to their very short growth cycle [8], industrial materials such as bioplastics and production of biohydrogen [9], alternative biological agents in wastewater treatment [10] and so forth, which would be discussed in other chapters.

This chapter will focus on the current applications as well as prospective use of those algal biocompounds in humans, further divided into three sections according to the application of the biocompounds, namely dietary, cosmetical and pharmaceutical uses. The common algae species for each of the applications will also be discussed.

## 2. Dietary use as food supplements and additives

In an era where sustainable and nutritious food solutions are essential, algae have emerged as a promising resource for both food supplements and additives. These diverse aquatic organisms, ranging from microscopic microalgae to large seaweeds, are rich in valuable nutrients and bioactive compounds. Their unique advantages, particularly their rapid growth and short lifecycles, position algae as one of the key contributors to addressing global challenges related to food security and health. This section will explore the various applications of algae and their biocompounds in the food industry.

## 2.1 Food supplements

Food supplements are concentrated nutrients that are essential or beneficial to the human body. They are usually in the form of pills, tablets, capsules or liquids, depending on their inherited characteristics, and are designed to be easy and convenient for consumption. Legally, they are situated in between food and medicine and are usually regulated as food in many countries, for example in the European Union. Algae and microalgae, demonstrated to possess diverse health benefits, together with the fact that they are generally recognized as safe for their long history as food, are one of the major sources of food supplements nowadays.

Currently, commercialized microalgal products are presented in many forms. They are sometimes marketed as health food alone, usually in the forms of tablets, capsules and liquids [11]; or the algae and/or their extracts could be blended into different foods such as pastes, snacks, candy, noodles, beverages, breakfast cereals, etc. [12–14]. To date, *Spirulina sp.* and *Chlorella sp.* remain the most widely used algal species in food, along with a few other species such as *Aphanizomenon flosaquae*, *Dunaliella salina* and *Dunaliella tertiolecta* [3].

### *2.1.1 Source of macronutrients*

The first generation of algae-based food supplements, developed during the mid-twentieth century food crisis, primarily focused on providing macronutrients such as proteins and fatty acids [15]. Algae possess a competitive advantage of fast and cost-effective photosynthetic growth, primarily due to their capability to be grown in high biomass concentration. This trail greatly boosts the overall solar-to-biomass conversion efficiency in some strains of algae and results in a 16-fold increase in biomass when compared to terrestrial corn grown in the same amount of land [16]. Another study by Ullah et al. even found that algae can produce a maximum of about 160 times biomass more than corn, despite being in very confined conditions [17].

On top of normal biomass, many algae species are found capable of yielding very high levels of desired nutrients under cultivation. *Chlorella* spp., one of the most widely cultivated species, was reported to produce a maximum of about 65% of protein in dry weight [18]. *Spirulina* spp., another commonly harvested algae nowadays, on the other hand yet similarly, had been found to have a maximum protein level of 60–70% in dry weight, significantly higher than all common meat and fish (by contrast, beef contains about 22% protein in dry weight) [19]. Further, unlike most of the ordinary plant-based proteins, proteins derived from algae have a comprehensive profile thanks to the presence of both essential and non-essential amino acids in sufficient quantities.

In addition, the role of algae in food production, especially for protein, is becoming increasingly prominent in the current era of climate change. Currently, the livestock supply chain – the traditional protein production – alone accounts for about 14.5% of total greenhouse gas emissions worldwide [20], because of its inefficient energy transfer across three trophic levels. Contrastingly, being an autotroph, algal-based proteins are comparingly much sustainable, and the proteins are foreseen to be one of the major players in alternative protein production in the near future [21].

Despite all these outstanding features, algae do have limitations that hinder commercialization as a major food source. The greatest obstacle is the unreasonably high cost of harvesting, which alone could account for up to 30% of total production cost, due to high energy demand and capital cost. Common harvesting methods at the time involved filtration, centrifugation, flocculation, and flotation, or a combination of the above methods [22]. It was only with technological advancements and cost reductions since the 1960s that microalgal products began to be used as food supplements worldwide.

Amazingly, microalgae species can be engineered the other way around to have relatively low protein levels while being high in lipid content. Unlike typical macroalgae seaweed that contains only 2–4.5% of lipids (in the form of glycolipids and phospholipids) in their dry weight, microalgae could be manipulated to contain from around 20–50% to as high as 80% of lipids, under specific and optimized culturing conditions [22]. The main drawback of algal lipid production maybe its high water consumption, with an estimated requirement of over 3700 kg of water for every 1 kg of lipid produced. The huge consumption, however, could be reduced significantly, as 90% of wastewater produced could be recycled for algae cultivation [23]. Currently, algal lipids are primarily used for oil or biodiesel production, rather than for human consumption and applications discussed in this chapter.

Despite the absence of commercial dietary supplements solely based on algal lipids, algae, especially microalgae, were found to produce various forms of essential fatty acids, such as Omega-3 and Omega-6 including the most popular and widely commercialized eicosapentaenoic acid (EPA) and docosahexaenoic acid (DHA), alongside with linoleic acid, gamma-linolenic acid, arachidonic acid, and more [24]. These fatty acids are well-known for significantly enhancing human health by lowering the possibility of cardiovascular diseases and hypertension, inflammation regulation, and brain development, just to name a few. Microalgae such as *Nannochloropsis* spp., *Tetraselmis* spp. and some others are capable of mass producing such essential fatty acids for human consumption in a relatively large quantity and sustainable manner [25].

#### *2.1.2 Source of micronutrients*

More than macronutrients, algae were found to contain abundantly many types of micronutrients like vitamins and minerals. For instance, studies showed that microalgae were excellent sources of vitamins (A, B1, B2, B12, C and E), iodine, potassium, iron, magnesium and calcium [3]. However, to the best effort of the author, there is no standalone commercial micronutrient supplement on the market advertised as being naturally extracted from algae. All these products are marketed as whole algae that contain rich amounts of advertised micronutrients. This is probably because of the relatively high price of purifying such micronutrients and the availability of alternative inexpensive sources elsewhere.

### 2.2 Food additives

#### *2.2.1 Colourings*

Algae serve as a valuable source of natural food colourings, with chlorophylls, carotenoids, and phycobiliproteins being the most commonly used additives in the food industry.

Chlorophylls are a group of green pigments naturally produced by various types of both macroalgae and microalgae for photosynthesis, alongside many terrestrial plants. Contrary to their biological function of absorbing photons, purified chlorophylls are surprisingly rather unstable and easily degraded by light, acid, base and oxidants. In order to maintain their colour stably, food industries often use chlorophyllide, a slightly modified form of chlorophyll, as a colouring agent [26]. While almost all plants contain chlorophyll, algae especially *Spirulina* spp., contain much higher content of chlorophylls (a and b), up to three times that of other plants [27], rendering them an economic source of chlorophylls for production of chlorophyllide in the industry.

Carotenoids are a diverse group of approximately 500 unsaturated hydrocarbons that frequently serve as accessory pigments in the light-harvesting process within chloroplasts [28]. They are widely presented in many algal taxa in high amounts, for instance, *Chlorophyta, Rhodophyta, Phaeophyta, Dinoflagellate* [29]. Carotenoids supplement chlorophylls and hence strongly absorb wavelengths they leave behind, that is, 400–600 nm, and thus appear red to yellow in colour. Common carotenoids that are isolated from algae include β-carotene, astaxanthin, lutein and zeaxanthin, and all of them have high potential to be used as food colourings. However, carotenoids extracted from algae have not yet been widely used nowadays due to their stability and technological constraints [26].

Phycobiliproteins are another very important photosynthetic accessory pigments found commonly in blue-green algae (e.g., blue phycocyanin and light-blue allophycocyanin) and red algae (e.g., red phycoerythrobilin) [30]. Their bright colour and high yield make them another ideal colourings in the food industry. Most research to date focuses on the application of phycocyanin extracted from *Spirulina* spp., while phycobiliproteins from other algae also carry high potentials [31]. Notably, blue phycocyanin, among its other wide applications, is the only blue dye officially approved by the United States Food and Drug Administration (USFDA) to be used in foods and cosmetics [32]. Moreover, the proteins were also found to possess antioxidant, antiviral, anti-cancer, antiallergic, anti-inflammatory, and neuroprotective characteristics, with high potential to be further researched in healthcare applications [33]. The proteins' pharmaceutical functions will be further discussed in Section 4.

### 2.2.2 Thickeners

An important application of algae in the food industry is thickeners. Thickeners are defined by the USFDA as "substances used to produce viscous solutions or dispersions, to impart body, improve consistency, or stabilize emulsions" [34]. Polysaccharides extracted from macroalgae seaweeds are highly regarded by the industry as excellent thickeners, enhancing water absorption and texture in various products, including confectionery, dairy, desserts, bakery, meat and dressings [35]. The polysaccharides are mainly extracted from brown and red algae, and the polysaccharides commonly used include alginate (or algin), agar and carrageenan.

Alginates are a group of structurally similar copolymers composed of two main building blocks - mannuronic and guluronic acids. The ratio and distribution of the two blocks influence the physical properties of the alginate gel, such as its strength and elasticity. They are found in the cell walls of brown algae, enhancing their flexibility. Today, alginates are commonly extracted from brown algae including *Ascophyllum* spp., *Laminaria* spp., *Lessonia* spp. and *Macrocystis* spp. [28]. It was also reported that the alginate content increases in those algae that grow in more turbulent regions [36]. With its low gelation temperature, alginates are a popular choice of thickener in jam and pulp/paste in a wide variety of food. Nowadays, alginate is one of the most widely used thickeners in products for instance dairy and meat products [28].

Agar is another polysaccharide extracted from algae with similar functions as alginates. However, agar is extracted from the cell walls of red instead of brown algae. Common species suitable for extraction include *Gelidium* spp. and *Gracilaria* spp. [37]. While it may not affect too much the choice of food manufacturers, the most notable difference between agar and alginate is that the former is thermo-reversible whilst alginate is irreversible [38]. Likewise, agar is also widely applied in diverse types of food, for example, dairy products (e.g., cheese, cream, milk deserts, yoghurt), cereal-based products and even some meat products [37].

Carrageenan is a family of linear sulfated polysaccharides with molecular sizes between 200 and 800 kDa [39]. Commercially, three types of carrageenan are commonly used, namely κ-Carrageenan (Kappa), ι-Carrageenan (Iota) and λ-Carrageenan (Lambda) [40]. They are regarded as 'Generally Recognized as Safe' in both the United States and Europe and have been widely used in commercialized food such as ice creams, chocolate milk, pudding, condensed milk and more. More than thickeners, carrageenan is also used as a gelling, water-holding, stabilizing, and emulsifying agent in the food industry. Recently, their potential use in mimicking meat products by binding meat-free ingredients for vegetarians is also explored [39]. The multi-purpose polysaccharides could be extracted from a variety of red algae for instance *Kappaphycus alvarezii*, *Eucheuma denticulatum*, *Chondrus crispus* and *Sarcothalia crispate* [41].

### *2.2.3 Prebiotics*

Prebiotics are food substances that resist digestion in the upper gastrointestinal tract. These non-digestible substances then reach the lower tract particularly the colon where they are selectively fermented by beneficial gut bacteria, like bifido-bacteria and lactobacilli [42]. The fermentation process promotes the growth and activity of these beneficial microflora, leading to the production of short-chain fatty acids like butyrate, acetate and propionate. These fatty acids in return provide various health benefits, including improved gut barrier function, reduced inflammation and modulation of the immune system [43]. Algal products are gaining recognition as promising prebiotics due to the presence of unique non-digestible polysaccharides. These polysaccharides are present in many algae in high quantities. With many of them under intense research, a few polysaccharides were recognized scientifically for their activity, which include galacto-oligosaccharides, agar or agarose-derived oligosaccharides, xylo-oligosaccharides, alginate-derived oligosaccharides [44]. The incorporation of algal products into the diet can therefore serve as a natural strategy to support a healthy gut microbiota and overall well-being.

## 3. External use as cosmetics

Cosmetics are defined as articles intended to be applied to the human body, for various aesthetic purposes, including cleansing, beautifying, promoting attractive-ness or altering the appearance. They could also be applied to the human body by various methods such as rubbing, pouring, sprinkling spraying, etc. [45]. Many algae species contain biocompounds with beneficial cosmetic properties and are used in cosmetic products. Historically used for thousands of years, algae are considered generally safe with minimal cytotoxicity to humans [46]. Additionally, the use of algal ingredients in cosmetics perfectly aligns with the current trend of naturalness in human use of bioproducts [47], and is often heavily advertised today by various brands.

The vast amount of different bioactive compounds had been successfully isolated from various algae suitable for cosmetical use, with examples including polysaccharides, sulfated polysaccharides, pigments, polyphenols, phenolic compounds, bioactive peptides, proteins, mycosporine-like amino acids, etc., [48]. In Europe alone, at least 29 patents related to algae-based cosmetics were filed between 2010 and 2023 showcasing various solutions for different skin concerns [49]. Cosmetical uses of macroalgae and microalgae ingredients can be categorized into seven major categories, including anti-aging, moisturizing, whitening, thickening, photoprotection and antioxidant and hair care [48].

### 3.1 Anti-aging

Aging is a complicated and multicausal phenomenon, exacerbated by extrinsic factors such as UV radiation, air pollution and smoking. It eventually results in the deterioration of skin cells which manifest dryness, dull, uneven and wrinkled [48]. Given that algae in the ocean are naturally exposed to UV radiation and oxidative stress, many bioactive compounds extracted therein, for example, polysaccharides, sulfated galactan, sulfated galactofucans, peptides, polyunsaturated fatty acid, fucoxanthine, mycosporine-like amino acids and astaxanthin were found to possess anti-oxidative and anti-aging properties [50].

Fucoidan, a type of sulfated polysaccharide primarily derived from brown algae, exhibits a range of bioactivities and deserves special attention. For instance, the fucoidan extracted from *Fucus vesiculosus* has been incorporated into skin care products and shown to possess anti-aging and anti-wrinkle benefits. The study suggested that the fucoidan worked by enhancing dermal fibroblast proliferation and therefore promoting collagen production [48]. Moreover, another research also showed that fucoidan extract can reduce dark circles beneath the eye, possibly by accelerating the removal of heme catabolites through upregulating the rate-limiting heme oxygenase activity [51]. The polysaccharides were also demonstrated to exhibit various other beneficial effects depending on their molecular weight and sulphation, such as antitumour, antioxidant, anti-coagulant, anti-thrombotic, immunomodulatory, antiviral and anti-inflammatory. In addition to *F. vesiculosus*, fucoidan has also been reported in various other species of brown algae, such as *Dictyota* spp., *Ascophyllum nodosum, and Sargassum cymosum* [52].

Many research groups also have reported numerous other anti-aging biocompounds that have yet to be isolated and analyzed. Most of them only reported relatively preliminary results that anti-aging biocompounds were present in either water- or organic-soluble extracts from a wide variety of different algae. Those algae concerned included *Ahnfeltiopsis* spp., *Chlorococcum* spp., *Colpomenia* spp., *Halymenia* spp., *Gracilaria* spp., *Hydroclathrus* spp., *Kappaphycus* spp., *Laurencia* spp., *Macrocystis* spp., *Nannochloropsis* spp., *Nostoc* spp., *Polysiphonia* spp., *Padina* spp., *Turbinaria* spp., just to name a few [48].

### 3.2 Whitening

White skin, or lighter skin colour, is commonly regarded as beauty and highly desirable, especially among women in Asian, African and Caribbean countries. It was estimated that the global market for skin whitening products will almost double from USD$ 8.8 billion in 2022 to more than 15 billion in 2030 [53], with another more ambitious estimate that it could reach as much as 31.2 billion by 2024 [54].

One of the most common approaches for skin whitening commercially, also known as skin bleaching, involves the inhibition of the copper-containing tyrosinase enzyme, thereby reducing melanin synthesis, that is, the natural dark biological pigment that gives colour, in melanocytes inside human skin. The reduction of dark pigment eventually makes the skin look whiter and lighter.

A few categories of bioactive compounds extracted from algae were shown to possess skin whitening capability. For instance, polysaccharides and their degradation products from three red algae species (*Porphyra haitanensis, Gracilaria chouae* and *Gracilaria blodgettii*) [55] and another three species of seaweed from genus *Sargassum* [48], bromophenols from another species of red algae (*Odonthalia corymbifera*) [56], polyphenols from brown algae *Padina boryana* [57] and fucosterol from *Padina gymnospora* [58] were also found to possess similar tyrosinase inhibitory capability. It is worth noting that zeaxanthin, initially extracted from the microalgae *Nannochloropsis oculata*, has been used in cosmetic whitening creams available on the market in the past decade [59]. The zeaxanthin could also be isolated from other microalgae, for example, some blue-green algae and red algae, in high yield [60].

### 3.3 Moisturizing

Moisturizers are a group of cosmetics that maintain, and better improve, the barrier function of the skin, thereby keeping its healthy appearance. Medically, they are compounds that are capable of increasing skin hydration through reducing trans-epidermal water loss from the skin surface, commonly by holding water *in-situ* or forming a layer of impermeable film to counteract evaporation [61].

Algae are rich in polysaccharides and oligosaccharides which are excellent in storing water, at the same time connecting to the skin keratin with hydrogen bonds [49]. Polysaccharides differ in weight and functional groups, which in turn affects their moisturizing properties. The sulfated polysaccharides isolated from a red alga (*Porphyra* spp.) were found to improve the maturation of the keratinized envelope and possess a strong and prolonged moisturizing effect [62]. On the other hand, lipid molecules extracted from brown macroalgae *Laminaria ochroleuca* contain up to 55% unsaturated fatty acids that help to regulate trans-epidermal water loss. The fatty acids were proven for their excellent moisturizing properties and are widely used in commercial skincare products [63].

### 3.4 Thickening

Similar to thickeners in food industries, the extracts from various geniuses of algae, mainly the polysaccharides alginate, agar and carrageenan mentioned in the previous section, could be incorporated into cosmetic formulations as a thickening agent in notions, creams, bath soap/rinse, lipsticks [7]. The algae-derived thickeners are also often marketed as natural, sustainable, and skin-friendly, distinguishing them from their counterpart which are made synthetically [48].

### 3.5 Photoprotection and antioxidant

Human skin is prone to damage by excessive exposure to sunlight due to the generation of reactive oxygen species, damaging DNA or other cellular components, and resulting in diverse skin problems for instance hyperpigmentation, dullness, lack of radiance, uneven skin tone, wrinkles and more [64]. Screening of ultraviolet radiation could therefore effectively avoid such damage. Furthermore, unlike mainstream chemical sunscreen using titanium and zinc oxides that cause marine pollution and intoxication, algal products are easily biodegraded and cause no harm to the environment [65]. Microalgal compounds can protect human skin through three mechanisms, either individually or in combination: first, by directly screening UV rays, second, by scavenging free radicals generated by UV exposure and third, by protecting skin cells from damage caused by these radicals [66].

Microalgae are known to produce numerous photoprotective and anti-oxidative biocompounds, for example, mycosporine-like amino acids produced by a range of algal species such as *Aphanizomenon flos-aquae*. The small acids are capable of absorbing and thereby screening UV radiation between 310 and 360 nm from the skin [67]. Moreover, biocompounds from many other algal species, such as carotenoid, astaxanthin, phenolic compounds (e.g., phlorotannins) and polyunsaturated fatty acids were also shown to have antioxidant and photoprotection properties [68, 69]. Another study conducted by Mercurio et al. using immunohistochemical analysis also confirmed that extracts from a red alga *Porphyra umbilicalis* exhibited strong cell protection against DNA damage caused by ultraviolet A (UVA) radiation in mice, and hence considered an excellent alternative ingredient in sunscreen formulation [70], just to name a few. In a recent study, it was found that the extract of a green microalga *Tetraselmis suecica* contains a cocktail of carotenoids. The carotenoids were found capable of promoting cellular repair in reconstructed human epidermal tissue cells damaged by hydrogen peroxide treatment [71]. Today, some of the biocompounds have been adopted commercially by several companies, mostly being one of the alternative active ingredients in sunscreen products, which can provide protection up to the level of SPF 50 [66].

### 3.6 Hair care

The perseverance of full-head hair is getting more important, especially for males in their middle of age. Androgenetic alopecia, commonly known as hair loss disorder, is becoming not only a dermatological problem but also, if not more frustrating, a psychological nightmare. The causes of hair loss are often linked to direct contact of chemicals such as air pollutants with the hair dermis, alongside a cocktail of many other factors, including inherent genetic makeup. The root cause is often difficult to diagnose and singled out [72].

For centuries, ancient societies believed that consuming brown algae could enhance hair health. Algal ingredients primarily support hair care by protecting hair follicles. For example, studies demonstrated that algal extracts could help prevent hair loss through enzymatic and anti-inflammatory activities [73], as well as regulating androgen-induced growth factors [74]. *Ex-vivo* experiments from another group using mice further confirmed that the extracts from two edible brown algae possess the same hair growth effect as a typical hair loss medication (i.e., 3% minoxidil) [75]. Microalgal extracts selectively extracted using solvents from *Monodus* spp., *Thalassiosira* spp., *Chaetoceros* spp. and *Chlorococcum* spp. were already patented for cosmetics use with their outstanding properties in modulating the metabolism of human skin and hair follicles [76].

Notably, other ingredients extracted from algae, for instance, vitamin E and carotene, are often incorporated into the formula to maximize protection and healing. Today, algal extracts are marketed in some middle to high-end hair care brands, including Revlon (US), Onsensou (Japan), Nanoil (US), Mielle (P&G) and so fore.

## 4. Pharmaceutical use

Algal biocompounds are shown to provide various benefits in humans and have a high potential to be used as pharmaceuticals. Among them, some possess potent effects and/or multiple functions that with high prospects to be further developed for disease curing. These compounds have various therapeutic functions such as anti-microbial, anti-inflammatory, hypertension management, anti-cancer and aid and clinical diagnosis (**Table 1**). This section will explore some promising applications of algal biocompounds nowadays.

| Application | Target subject | Bioproduct category | Active algal bioproduct(s) | Common algae (group/strain) |
|---|---|---|---|---|
| Anti-virus | HIV | Polysaccharides | Sulfated polymannuro-guluronate | Brown algae [77] |
| | HIV | | Galactan sulfate | Red algae *Agardhiella tenera* [78] |
| | HIV | | Griffithsin | Red algae *Griffithsia sp.* [78] |
| | Multiple (HIV, dengue virus, common cold virus, HPV) | | Carrageenan | Red algae [79] |
| | SARS-CoV-2 | | Fucoidans | *Saccharina japonica* [80] |
| Anti-bacteria | Common pathogens | Extract | — | Green algae *Scenedesmus obliquus* [81] |
| | Oral pathogens | Extract | Sulfated polysaccharide with some other chemicals | Green alga *Ulva lactuca* [24] |
| Antibacterial (aid to stabilize Ag NPs) | Gram + veand gram −ve bacteria | Polysaccharides | Sulfated polysaccharide | Green alga *Ulva armoricana* [82] |
| Anti-inflammation | — | — | Carotenoids (lutein and astaxanthin), fatty acid (EPA, DHA), mycosporine-like amino acids sulfated polysaccharides [28, 83] | Green algae and diatoms for example *Chlorella sp., Dunaliella sp., Phaeodactylum sp.,* etc. [84] |
| Hypertension management | Angiotensin-converting enzyme activity | Extract from supercritical carbon dioxide along with subcritical water extraction | Total flavonoid | Brown seaweed *Undaria pinnatifida* [85] |
| | Angiotensin -converting enzyme activity | Extract from sequential extraction | Hydrolyzed products from protein-polysaccharides | Brown seaweed *Saccharina latissima* and *Ascophyllum nodosum* [86] |
| Cancer treatment | Human breast cancer cell line (MCF7) | Polysaccharides | Porphyran | Red algae Ecklonia kurome [87] |

| Application | Target subject | Bioproduct category | Active algal bioproduct(s) | Common algae (group/ strain) |
|---|---|---|---|---|
| | Human breast cancer cell line (MCF7), colon cancer cell line (HT29), liver cancer cell line (HepG2) and osteosarcoma cell line (MG63) | | Carrageenan | Red algae *Kappaphycus alvarezii* [88] |
| | Human colon cancer cell line (HT29) and breast cancer cell line (T-47D) | | Fucoidan | Brown algae *Alaria marginata & Alaria angusta* [89] |
| | Mice (xenograft tumour and induced colorectal cancer models) | | β-1,3/1,6-glucan | Brown algae Durvillaea Antarctica [90] |
| | Human liver cancer cell line (HepG2), breast cancer cell line (MCF7) and cervical cancer cell line (HeLa) | | Ulvan | Green algae *Ulva lactuca* [91] |
| | Human colon cancer cell line (HT29) and HT-29 cell-xenograft nude mice | | Glucuronorhamnoxylan | Green algae *Capsosiphon fulvescens* [92] |
| | Breast cancer cell line (T47D) and colon cancer cell line (HT-29) | Extract (hexane fraction) | Fucosterol | Brown algae *Sargassum angustifolium* [93] |
| | ATM-deficient cell line (LoVo) and KB) | Others | Apratoxin | Blue-green algae *LYNGBYA sp.* [94] |
| | Human lung cancer cell line (A549) | | Curacin A | Blue-green algae *Lyngbya majuscula* [95] |
| | Murine leukaemia cells line (L1210) | | Cryptophycin 1 | Blue-green algae *Nostoc sp.* [96] |
| | Human breast cancer cell line (MCF7) | | Nigriccaoides A and B | Green algae *Avrainvillea nigricans* [97] |
| Cancer treatment (aids) | In-situ oxygenation | — | Whole algae | *Chlorella sp.* [98–100] |
| | Oral colon cancer drug delivery | — | Whole algae | Blue-green algae *Spirulina platensis* [101] |

| Application | Target subject | Bioproduct category | Active algal bioproduct(s) | Common algae (group/ strain) |
|---|---|---|---|---|
| Fluorescent dyes | Flow cytometry, fluorescence immuno-assay and microscopy | Extract (protein purified after cell disruption, isolation and chromato-graphic separation) | B-phycoerythrin | Red algae *Phorphyridium cruentum* [102] |
| | | | R-phycoerythrin | Red algae *Phorphyridium cruentum* [102] |
| | | | Allophycocyanin | Blue-green algae *Spirulina platensis* [102] |

**Table 1.**
*An overview of pharmaceutical applications of algae.*

## 4.1 Antimicrobial activities

### *4.1.1 Antiviral activities*

Seaweed, that is, macroalgae, the extract had long been reported to possess a protective effect against the virus [103]. Subsequent research found that the polysaccharides therein were responsible for the antiviral properties, with some of them were proven for obstructing the infection by Human Immunodeficiency Virus (HIV) such as alginate 911 [104], sulfated polymannuro-guluronate [77], a rhodophycean galactan sulfate [78] and so forth. Carrageenan, another group of very well-researched polysaccharides from red algae, exhibits potent antiviral effects not only on HIV but also against the dengue virus, human papillomavirus (HPV) and common cold virus [79]. The study reported that the polysaccharides were capable of both improving host immunity and suppressing the virus at the same time.

Apart from HIV, other research groups also showed that algal polysaccharides exhibit strong anti-influenza capabilities [105, 106], as well as the preventive and therapeutic capabilities against SARS-CoV-2 (COVID-19) infection [107]. Kwon et al. reported that the potent antiviral capability could be a result of the polysaccharides' exceptional binding affinity to the SARS-CoV-2's spike protein (S-protein). The group continued to propose that the two most potent polysaccharides, that is, fucoidans and trisulfated heparin, could be further researched and developed as nasal spray, inhaler or oral drug for infection treatment [80]. Moreover, the use of algae against SARS-CoV-2 virus extended beyond direct medication. There are also attempts to develop edible vaccines using genetically modified green microalgae (*Chlamydomonas reinhardtii)* to produce antibodies to combat the pandemic [108].

### *4.1.2 Antibacterial activities*

Unsurprisingly, algal extracts were also widely reported to possess antibacterial activities [109]. For example, extracts from a green alga *Scenedesmus obliquus* were shown to exhibit antibacterial activity against eight common pathogenic bacteria [81]. Likewise, extract from another green alga, *Ulva* spp. was reported to demonstrate antibacterial activity against oral pathogens. Nevertheless, their antibacterial activity could at best be rated as mild when compared to conventional antibiotics, and hence might not be a key candidate for next-generation antibiotics exploration [24]. Contrastingly, algal bioproducts stayed alive in the field as a treatment aid. A sulfated polysaccharide extracted from *Ulva* spp. was utilized as a stabilizer for silver nanoparticles, which together exhibited strong and fast antibacterial activities against both gram-positive and negative bacteria [82].

### 4.2 Anti-inflammatory

Algae, particularly microalgae, had been extensively shown to possess strong anti-inflammatory activity, alongside some other immunomodulatory properties. The activity has also been identified in a wide variety of green algae and diatoms, for example, *Chlorella* spp., *Dunaliella* spp., *Phaeodactylum* spp., etc. [84]. With the vast number of biocompounds involved, algal anti-inflammatory mechanisms are inevitably complex subjects to biocompounds involved. To date, isolated algal biocompounds found to have anti-inflammatory activity include carotenoids (lutein and astaxanthin), fatty acids (EPA, DHA), mycosporine-like amino acids and sulfated polysaccharides, etc. They were shown to counteracting a diverse type of inflammations from arthritis to autoimmune diseases [28, 83].

Clinically, whole algae supplement was also proven to possess anti-inflammatory activity. In medium-scale double-blind randomized trial with patients affected by non-alcoholic fatty liver disease, the group intervened with *Chlorella vulgaris* tablets was concluded to have significantly lower serum levels of the pro-inflammatory cytokine TNF-$\alpha$, a biomarker that induces inflammation [110].

### 4.3 Mediation for hypertension

There are reports that extract from a brown seaweed *Undaria pinnatifida* possesses anti-hypertensive activities, which has the potential for use as a medication to lower blood pressure. The group also discovered that the activity was linked to the total flavonoid content levels, based on their correlation analysis [85]. Another group experimenting on another two brown algae *Saccharina latissima* and *Ascophyllum nodosum* speculated that the activity could be a result of protein-polysaccharides conjugates. When hydrolyzed, the short peptides target the angiotensin I-converting enzyme, thereby inhibiting the formation of angiotensin II [86].

It is noteworthy that other bioproducts from algae, for example, omega-3 fatty acids, antioxidants, etc., could also assist in lowering blood pressure indirectly by suppressing inflammation. Algae are also a source of both soluble and insoluble dietary fibre, which helps lower blood pressure by slowing down digestion and thus glucose absorption. There is also evidence that dietary fibre promotes fermentation that led to the production of short-chain fatty acids, which were clinically linked to a reduction in hypertension [111].

### 4.4 Cancer prevention or curing

Cancer prevention and curing from biocompounds isolated from algae is one of the most researched areas in the field. Decades of efforts resulted in more than a hundred such biocompounds being isolated and assayed using various different cancer cell lines (and sometimes *in vivo*) around the world. For example, in blue-green algae, potent anti-cancer biocompounds like apratoxin ($LC_{50}$ of 0.36–0.52 nM from *Lyngbya sp.*), curacin A ($LC_{50}$ of <1 ug/mL from *Lyngbya majuscule*) and Cryptophycin 1 ($LC_{50}$ of 1 uM from *Nostoc sp.*) were isolated and tested. Likewise in green algae, anti-cancer biocompounds like nigriccaoides A and B ($LC_{50}$ of 3 nM from *Avrainvillea nigricans*) and Lycopene ($LC_{50}$ of 1–2 uM from *Chlorella zofingiensis*) had been found and assayed. Some less potent anti-cancer biocompounds can also be isolated from red and brown algae [112].

Polysaccharides are another group comprising of diverse anti-cancer biocompounds that worth particular attention. Yao and others found that almost a dozen of polysaccharides, e.g. porphyran, carrageenan, sulfated galactan, fucoidan, laminaran, β-1,3/1,6-glucan, fucan, ulvan and sulfated glucuronorhamnoxylan, exert potent anticancer effects against different cancer cell lines. The group further summarized that there are at least seven mechanisms involved, namely cell proliferation inhibition, apoptosis, cell cycle arrest, angiogenesis and metastasis inhibition, reactive oxygen species scavenging, immune response incitation and gut microbiota regulation [113].

Another potential candidate is fucosterol which is a water-insoluble steroid with a molecular weight of 412.7 ($C_{29}H_{48}O$). It is found commonly in brown macroalgae. Today, the steroid is mainly isolated from *Sargassum* spp., for example, *S. angustifolium*. It was reported to possess various beneficial physiological activities such as antioxidant, anti-inflammatory, anti-depressant, anti-aging, antidiabetic, cholesterol-lowering, among many others, in different *in-vitro* and *in-vivo* models [114]. In particular, there is a high potential that fucosterol could be developed as an anticancer drug with its potent inhibitory and cytotoxic effects against various cancer cell lines, for example, breast cancer, colon cancer, cervical cancer and lung cancer cells [115]. In a recent study, potent anti-cancer effect was observed whilst damage against normal cells was weak if not nominal. The group found that the steroid killed the cancer cells not only by inducing apoptosis, but also by downregulating essential cell cycle proteins to trigger $G_2$/M cell cycle arrest. Similar effects were observed in their further experiment using mice as subjects, that the growth of the xenografted tumours was inhibited [116].

However, despite several anti-cancer biocompounds being identified, their clinical application as anti-cancer drugs are still in its infancy stage as most of the studies involved *in-vitro* and *in-vivo* only. To the best effort of the author, no approved anticancer drug available today is isolated from algae. They are hence more likely a functional food to prevent cancers [117] rather than a marketable pharmaceutical at this moment. Furthermore, and especially for polysaccharides, given the wide diversity of isomers present, more systematic research on each of them is required.

### 4.5 Aid in cancer therapies

Further to being developed as a drug to directly cure cancer, algae could also be used as aids in cancer therapy in a number of ways. Whereas hypoxia is a state that confers tumour tolerance and promotes invasion and metastasis, microalgae, on the other hand, are of high photosynthetic efficiency which enables them to continuously produce oxygen using carbon dioxide if a photon of the desired wavelength is provided. They are hence excellent candidates to be used for local oxygenation, providing a source of reactive oxygen for highly oxygen-dependent treatments such as radiation therapy and photodynamic therapy, thereby improving the effectiveness of those treatments [118]. In fact, some groups have already developed prototypes using live *Chlorella sp*. to alleviate hypoxia and curing the cancer, with encouraging outcomes in animal models [98–100].

Algae can, at the same time, be utilized as a targeted drug delivery system for cancer therapy, alongside other various diseases. Inherently, algae show strong adsorption to a variety of compounds, and their surface could be easily modified to aid drug delivery [119]. For example, the blue-green algae *Spirulina* is ideal for drug loading and cargo transport given their hollow microhelical structure. With their spiral structure that enhances attachment to intestinal villi, a group proved that the *Spirulina platensis* could act as an excellent transporter to cure colon cancer. Notably, the transporter (plus an approved anti-cancer drug) was designed to be administered orally which added much flexibility to intestinal cancer therapy. Moreover, the transporter concurrently exerted concurrently anti-inflammatory effects against colitis during the treatment [101]. Another group demonstrated that, with magnetic actuation, microswimmers synthesized using the same algae achieved both high tumour accumulation potency as well as magnetic resonance imaging properties after intravenous injection. More importantly, the microswimmer system can itself act as a photosensitizer, which generates cytotoxic reactive oxygen species, to kill the cancer cells *in situ* [120]. Other similar magnetic delivery systems have also been developed recently, in which the same *Spirulina* species was incorporated into a nanomaterial microrobot to enhance its stability in aqueous dispersions and accumulation in cancer tissues. The microrobot achieved effective target cancer ablation and is capable of killing the cells in a short period of time [121].

### 4.6 Fluorescent dyes for clinical diagnosis and immunological analysis

Coloured algal pigments prominently phycobiliproteins could be purified for various clinical and immunological use. These proteins play a vital role in the photosynthetic process by supplementing light absorption in wavelengths where chlorophyll is not very efficient. They are hence found abundant in many types of algae, from blue-green algae to red algae to cryptomonads. Sekar and Chandramohan summarized the various categories of phycobiliproteins presented in algae in their review [102].

Phycobiliproteins are characterized by the number and structure of their chromophores called phycobilins which are attached to their polypeptide structure. Depending on the configuration of the chromophores, the protein can capture photons at the 450–650 nm range, giving them a high variety of colours and different absorption peaks for different applications [122]. Thanks to their natural involvement in the light-harvesting process, the group of proteins is reasonably stable and very soluble ideal for colorimetric use. They had been used as labels in immunoassay as early as the 1980s [123] and later marketed as diagnostic and laboratorial fluorescent dyes for more than a decade. Some commonly used and highly sensitive dyes include B-phycoerythrin, R-phycoerythrin and allophycocyanin.

Apart from clinical and immunological use, phycobiliproteins also possess multiple bioactivities such as antioxidant, antibacterial and anti-tumours, which makes them an excellent candidate in biochemical research. As discussed in Section 2, protein at the same time is an important colouring and attracted intense attention from the food and cosmetic industries [122]. According to a report from Future Market Insights, the market size of phycobiliprotein (phycocyanin) was expected to double from USD$ 754.40 million in 2022 to USD$1487.7 million in 2033 – a compound annual growth at about 7.3% [124].

## 5. Conclusion

In conclusion, this chapter has explored the multifaceted applications of algal biocompounds, demonstrating their significant potential across diverse sectors.

From their historical use as a food source to their modern applications in dietary supplements and additives, algae have proven to be a valuable resource of macro- and micronutrients, natural colourings, thickeners and prebiotics. Their unique nutritional profile, coupled with their sustainable cultivation potential, positions them as key players in addressing global food security and promoting healthy diets. Furthermore, the chapter highlighted the expanding role of algae in the cosmetic industry, where their bioactive compounds are utilized for anti-aging, whitening, moisturizing, photoprotection and hair care, aligning with the growing consumer demand for natural and sustainable beauty products. Finally, the chapter delved into the promising pharmaceutical applications of algal biocompounds, showcasing their antiviral, antibacterial and anti-inflammatory activities. They also show promise in hypertension management and anti-cancer therapies, both as direct treatments and as aids like targeted drug delivery. Algal pigments also serve as valuable fluorescent dyes in clinical analysis. These findings highlight algae's potential for future pharmaceutical development.

## Conflict of interest

The author declares no conflict of interest.

## Author details

Edwin H.W. Leung
University of Warwick, Coventry, United Kingdom

*Address all correspondence to: edwin.leung@warwick.ac.uk

## References

[1] Aaronson S. Algae. In: The Cambridge World History of Food. Cambridge: Cambridge University Press; 2000. pp. 231-249

[2] Moseley ME. The Maritime Foundations of Andean Civilization; 1975

[3] Sathasivam R, Radhakrishnan R, Hashem A, Abd Allah EF. Microalgae metabolites: A rich source for food and medicine. Saudi Journal of Biological Sciences. 2019;**26**:709-722

[4] García JL, de Vicente M, Galán B. Microalgae, old sustainable food and fashion nutraceuticals. Microbial Biotechnology. 2017;**10**:1017-1024

[5] AlFadhly NKZ, Alhelfi N, Altemimi AB, Verma DK, Cacciola F. tendencies affecting the growth and cultivation of genus spirulina: An investigative review on current trends. Plants. 2022;**11**:3063

[6] Laamanen CA, Desjardins SM, Senhorinho GNA, Scott JA. Harvesting microalgae for health beneficial dietary supplements. Algal Research. 2021;**54**:102189

[7] Ariede MB, Candido TM, Jacome ALM, Velasco MVR, de Carvalho JCM, Baby AR. Cosmetic attributes of algae - A review. Algal Research. 2017;**25**:483-487

[8] Zhou Y, Liu L, Li M, Hu C. Algal biomass valorisation to high-value chemicals and bioproducts: Recent advances, opportunities and challenges. Bioresource Technology. 2022;**344**:126371

[9] Calijuri ML, Silva TA, Magalhães IB, de Pereira ASAP, Marangon BB, de Assis LR, et al. Bioproducts from microalgae biomass: Technology, sustainability, challenges and opportunities. Chemosphere. 2022;**305**:135508

[10] Leung EHW, Lam W, Lo CM, Lee FWF, Xu SJL. Novel Nitrogen-Doped Zinc Oxide (ND-ZnO) Algal-Bioreactor System for Methylene Blue Wastewater Treatment. Journal of Environmental Engineering. 2024;**150**(2):04023102. DOI: 10.1061/JOEEDU.EEENG-7409

[11] Pulz O, Gross W. Valuable products from biotechnology of microalgae. Applied Microbiology and Biotechnology. 2004;**65**:635-648

[12] Lee Y-K. Commercial production of microalgae in the Asia-Pacific rim. Journal of Applied Phycology. 1997;**9**:403-411

[13] Liang S, Liu X, Chen F, Chen Z. Current microalgal health food R & D activities in China. In: Asian Pacific Phycology in the 21st Century: Prospects and Challenges. Netherlands, Dordrecht: Springer; 2004. pp. 45-48

[14] Yamaguchi K. Recent advances in microalgal bioscience in Japan, with special reference to utilization of biomass and metabolites: a review. Journal of Applied Phycology. 1996;**8**:487-502

[15] Vanhaute E. From famine to food crisis: what history can teach us about local and global subsistence crises. Journal of Peasant Studies. 2011;**38**:47-65

[16] Subramanian S, Sayre RT. The right stuff; realizing the potential for enhanced biomass production in microalgae. Frontiers in Energy Research. 2022;**10**. DOI: 10.3389/fenrg.2022.979747

[17] Ullah K, Ahmad M, Sofia SVK, Lu P, Harvey A, Zafar M, et al. Algal biomass

as a global source of transport fuels: Overview and development perspectives. Progress in Natural Science: Materials International. 2014;**24**:329-339

[18] Safafar H, Uldall Nørregaard P, Ljubic A, Møller P, Løvstad Holdt S, Jacobsen C. Enhancement of Protein and Pigment Content in Two Chlorella Species Cultivated on Industrial Process Water. Journal of Marine Science and Engineering. 2016;**4**:84

[19] AlFadhly NKZ, Alhelfi N, Altemimi AB, Verma DK, Cacciola F, Narayanankutty A. Trends and Technological Advancements in the Possible Food Applications of Spirulina and Their Health Benefits: A Review. Molecules. 2022;**27**:5584

[20] FAO. Livestock solutions for climate change. Rome: FAO; 2017. Available from: https://www.fao.org/family-farming/detail/en/c/1634679/

[21] Jareonsin S, Pumas C, Jaitiang D, Uttarotai T. Green fusion proteins: An approach to sustainable nutrition blending plant and algae-based proteins for a circular food system. Future Foods. 2024;**10**:100415

[22] Sen TJ, Lee SY, Chew KW, Lam MK, Lim JW, Ho S-H, et al. A review on microalgae cultivation and harvesting, and their biomass extraction processing using ionic liquids. Bioengineered. 2020;**11**:116-129

[23] Yang J, Xu M, Zhang X, Hu Q, Sommerfeld M, Chen Y. Life-cycle analysis on biodiesel production from microalgae: water footprint and nutrients balance. Bioresource Technology. 2011;**102**:159-165

[24] Kapoor DU, Kukkar MR, Gaur M, Prajapati BG, Suttiruengwong S, Sriamornsak P. Algae as third-generation materials: Exploring the emerging role in pharmaceutical applications. Materials Today Sustainability. 2024;**27**:100935

[25] Veerasamy V, Neethirajan V, SingarayarMS, BalasundaramD, DharmarP, Thilagar S. Microalgal biomass and lipid synergy for omega fatty acid enrichment: A sustainable source for food supplements & nutraceuticals. Algal Research. 2024;**80**:103514

[26] Chen Z, Wu W, Wen Y, Zhang L, Wu Y, Farid MS, et al. Recent advances of natural pigments from algae. Food Production, Processing and Nutrition. 2023;**5**:39

[27] Koh E-J, Kim K-J, Choi J, Kang D-H, Lee B-Y. Spirulina maxima extract prevents cell death through BDNF activation against amyloid beta 1-42 (Aβ 1-42) induced neurotoxicity in PC12 cells. Neuroscience Letters. 2018;**673**:33-38

[28] Singh M, Mal N, Trivedi D, Krishnamoorthy S, Behera C, Krishnan C, et al. An overview of the role of algae-fortified foods in nutraceutical industries: Synthesis pathway of value-added bioproducts and co-products. Food Bioscience. 2025;**63**:105568

[29] Takaichi S. Carotenoids in Algae: Distributions, Biosyntheses and Functions. Marine Drugs. 2011;**9**:1101-1118

[30] Imchen T, Singh KS. Marine algae colorants: Antioxidant, anti-diabetic properties and applications in food industry. Algal Research. 2023;**69**:102898

[31] Minić S, Gligorijević N, Veličković L, Nikolić M. Narrative Review of the Current and Future Perspectives of Phycobiliproteins' Applications in the Food Industry: From Natural Colors to Alternative Proteins. International Journal of Molecular Sciences. 2024;**25**:7187

[32] Najar-Almanzor CE, Velasco-Iglesias KD, Nunez-Ramos R,

Uribe-Velázquez T, Solis-Bañuelos M, Fuentes-Carrasco OJ, et al. Microalgae-assisted green bioremediation of food-processing wastewater: A sustainable approach toward a circular economy concept. Journal of Environmental Management. 2023;**345**:118774

[33] Chew KW, Yap JY, Show PL, Suan NH, Juan JC, Ling TC, et al. Microalgae biorefinery: High value products perspectives. Bioresource Technology. 2017;**229**:53-62

[34] FDA. Food Additives. United States; 2004. Available from: https://www.ecfr.gov/current/title-21/chapter-I/subchapter-B/part-170

[35] Malafronte L, Yilmaz-Turan S, Krona A, Martinez-Sanz M, Vilaplana F, Lopez-Sanchez P. Macroalgae suspensions prepared by physical treatments: Effect of polysaccharide composition and microstructure on the rheological properties. Food Hydrocolloids. 2021;**120**:106989

[36] Pradhan B, Ki J-S. Seaweed-derived laminarin and alginate as potential chemotherapeutical agents: An updated comprehensive review considering cancer treatment. International Journal of Biological Macromolecules. 2024:136593

[37] Ayyakkalai B, Nath J, Rao HG, Venkata V, Nori SS, Suryanarayan S. Seaweed derived sustainable packaging. In: Applications of Seaweeds in Food and Nutrition. Netherlands: Elsevier HQ; 2024. pp. 263-287

[38] Cervino G, Fiorillo L, Herford AS, et al. Alginate Materials and Dental Impression Technique: A Current State of the Art and Application to Dental Practice. Marine Drugs. 2018;**17**:18

[39] Udo T, Mummaleti G, Mohan A, Singh RK, Kong F. Current and emerging applications of carrageenan in the food industry. Food Research International. 2023;**173**:113369

[40] FAO. Production and Utilization of Products from Commercial Seaweeds. Rome: FAO; 1987. Available from: https://www.fao.org/4/x5822e/x5822e00.htm

[41] Naseri A, Holdt SL, Jacobsen C. Biochemical and Nutritional Composition of Industrial Red Seaweed Used in Carrageenan Production. Journal of Aquatic Food Product Technology. 2019;**28**:967-973

[42] Gotteland M, Riveros K, Gasaly N, Carcamo C, Magne F, Liabeuf G, et al. The Pros and Cons of Using Algal Polysaccharides as Prebiotics. Frontiers in Nutrition. 2020;**7**. DOI: 10.3389/fnut.2020.00163

[43] Silva YP, Bernardi A, Frozza RL. The Role of Short-Chain Fatty Acids From Gut Microbiota in Gut-Brain Communication. Frontiers in Endocrinology. 2020;**11**. DOI: 10.3389/fendo.2020.00025

[44] De Jesus RM, De Morais A, De Morais R. Emergent Sources of Prebiotics: Seaweeds and Microalgae. Marine Drugs. 2016;**14**:27

[45] Food and Drug Administration. FD&C Act. United States; 2018

[46] Thiyagarasaiyar K, Goh B-H, Jeon Y-J, Yow Y-Y. Algae Metabolites in Cosmeceutical: An Overview of Current Applications and Challenges. Marine Drugs. 2020;**18**:323

[47] Lunardo R, Saintives C. The effect of naturalness claims on perceptions of food product naturalness in the point of purchase. Journal of Retailing and Consumer Services. 2013;**20**:529-537

[48] Saini KC, Rani A, Gupta SK, Sharma P. Algae a Potential Source in Cosmetics: Current Status, Challenges, and Economic Implications. Indian Journal of Microbiology. 2024;**64**: 1445-1460. DOI: 10.1007/s12088-024-01263-0

[49] Hernández Muñoz AC, Rodríguez Martínez IA, Serafini MR, Aragón DM. Innovative applications of marine-derived algae in cosmetics: A patent review (2010–2023). Algal Research. 2024;**84**:103806

[50] Michalak I, Dmytryk A, Chojnacka K. Algae Cosmetics. In: Encyclopedia of Marine Biotechnology. New Jersey, US: Wiley; 2020. pp. 65-85

[51] Sun Y, Chavan M. Cosmetic Compositions Comprising Marine Plants; 2017

[52] Anjana K, Arunkumar K. Brown algae biomass for fucoxanthin, fucoidan and alginate; update review on structure, biosynthesis, biological activities and extraction valorisation. International Journal of Biological Macromolecules. 2024;**280**:135632

[53] Arora N, Amin S. Analyzing Global Interest in Skin Whitening by Geographic Region. Baylor University Medical Center Proceedings. 2024;**37**:505-507

[54] Zhao W, Yang A, Wang J, et al. Potential application of natural bioactive compounds as skin-whitening agents: A review. Journal of Cosmetic Dermatology. 2022;**21**:6669-6687

[55] Xie X-T, Zhang X, Liu Y, Chen X-Q, Cheong K-L. Quantification of 3,6-anhydro-galactose in red seaweed polysaccharides and their potential skin-whitening activity. 3 Biotech. 2020;**10**:189

[56] Islam MR, Mikami D, Kurihara H. Tyrosinase inhibitory and antioxidant activity by bromophenols from the alga Odonthalia corymbifera. Natural Products an Indian Journal. 2017;**13**:110

[57] Jayawardena TU, Sanjeewa KKA, Kim H-S, Lee HG, Wang L, Lee D-S, et al. Padina boryana, a brown alga from the Maldives: inhibition of α-MSH-stimulated melanogenesis via the activation of ERK in B16F10 cells. Fisheries and Aquatic Science. 2020;**23**:8

[58] Kim HK, Bak J, Kang HB, Kim M-J, Kim J-M, Min K, et al. The Skin-Whitening Effects of Padina Gymnospora and Its Active Compound, Fucosterol. Journal of Life Sciences. 2020;**30**:598-605

[59] Babitha S, Kim E-K. Effect of marine cosmeceuticals on the pigmentation of skin. Marine Cosmeceuticals: Trends and Prospects. 2011;**1**:63-66

[60] Bourdon L, Jensen AA, Kavanagh JM, McClure DD. Microalgal production of zeaxanthin. Algal Research. 2021;**55**:102266

[61] Draelos ZD. The science behind skin care: Moisturizers. Journal of Cosmetic Dermatology. 2018;**17**:138-144

[62] Zhang T, Guo Q, Xin Y, Liu Y. Comprehensive review in moisture retention mechanism of polysaccharides from algae, plants, bacteria and fungus. Arabian Journal of Chemistry. 2022;**15**:104163

[63] Otero P, López-Martínez MI, García-Risco MR. Application of pressurized liquid extraction (PLE) to obtain bioactive fatty acids and phenols from Laminaria ochroleuca collected in Galicia (NW Spain). Journal of Pharmaceutical and Biomedical Analysis. 2019;**164**:86-92

[64] Zhang T, Ungsurungsie M, Yue L, Li J, Zhuang B, Ding W, et al. Skin

photobiological effect induced by BL: Clinical manifestation, mechanisms, and protection against photodamages. Journal of Dermatologic Science and Cosmetic Technology. 2024;**1**:100042

[65] Lozano C, Givens J, Stien D, Matallana-Surget S, Lebaron P. Bioaccumulation and Toxicological Effects of UV-Filters on Marine Species; 2020, pp. 85-130

[66] Najafi A, Heidary M, Martinez RM, Baby AR, Morowvat MH. Microalgae-based sunscreens as green and sustainable cosmetic products. International Journal of Cosmetic Science. 2024. DOI: 10.1111/ics.13019

[67] Karsten U, Lembcke S, Schumann R. The effects of ultraviolet radiation on photosynthetic performance, growth and sunscreen compounds in aeroterrestrial biofilm algae isolated from building facades. Planta. 2007;**225**:991-1000

[68] Bedoux G, Hardouin K, Burlot AS, Bourgougnon N. Bioactive Components from Seaweeds; 2014, pp. 345-378

[69] Maadane A, Merghoub N, El Mernissi N, Ainane T, Amzazi S, Wahby I, et al. Antimicrobial activity of marine microalgae isolated from moroccan coastlines. Journal of Microbiology, Biotechnology and Food Sciences. 2017;**6**:1257-1260

[70] Mercurio DG, Wagemaker TAL, AlvesVM,BenevenutoCG,GasparLR,Maia Campos PMBG. In vivo photoprotective effects of cosmetic formulations containing UV filters, vitamins, Ginkgo biloba and red algae extracts. Journal of Photochemistry and Photobiology. B. 2015;**153**:121-126

[71] Sansone C, Galasso C, Orefice I, et al. The green microalga Tetraselmis suecica reduces oxidative stress and induces repairing mechanisms in human cells. Scientific Reports. 2017;**7**:41215

[72] Aggarwal A, Gupta R, Thukral N, Nandi G, Bora G. Analysis of various factors responsible for hair loss and awareness level in Delhi and the National Capital Region of India. Current Science. 2020;**118**:786-791

[73] Aslam A, Bahadar A, Liaquat R, Saleem M, Waqas A, Zwawi M. Algae as an attractive source for cosmetics to counter environmental stress. Science of the Total Environment. 2021;**772**:144905

[74] Huang C-Y, Huang C-Y, Yang C-C, Lee T-M, Chang J-S. Hair growth-promoting effects of Sargassum glaucescens oligosaccharides extracts. Journal of the Taiwan Institute of Chemical Engineers. 2022;**134**:104307

[75] Park KS, Park DH. Comparison of Saccharina japonica–Undaria pinnatifida mixture and minoxidil on hair growth promoting effect in mice. Archives of Plastic Surgery. 2016;**43**:498-505

[76] Zanella L, Pertile P, Massironi M, Massironi M, Caviola E. Extracts of Microalgae and their Application; 2018

[77] Meiyu G, Fuchuan L, Xianliang X, Jing L, Zuowei Y, Huashi G. The potential molecular targets of marine sulfated polymannuroguluronate interfering with HIV-1 entry Interaction between SPMG and HIV-1 rgp120 and CD4 molecule. Antiviral Research. 2003;**59**:127-135

[78] Yasuhara-Bell J, Lu Y. Marine compounds and their antiviral activities. Antiviral Research. 2010;**86**:231-240

[79] Grassauer A, Weinmuellner R, Meier C, Pretsch A, Prieschl-Grassauer E, Unger H. Iota-Carrageenan is a potent inhibitor of rhinovirus infection. Virology Journal. 2008;**5**:107

[80] Kwon PS, Oh H, Kwon S-J, Jin W, Zhang F, Fraser K, et al. Sulfated polysaccharides effectively inhibit SARS-CoV-2 in vitro. Cell Discover. 2020;**6**:50

[81] Bastia AK. In vitro antioxidant and antibacterial activity of Scenedesmus obliquus collected from Similipal biosphere reserve, Odisha, India. Journal of Indian Botanical Society. 2022;**102**:218-228

[82] Massironi A, Morelli A, Grassi L, Puppi D, Braccini S, Maisetta G, et al. Ulvan as novel reducing and stabilizing agent from renewable algal biomass: Application to green synthesis of silver nanoparticles. Carbohydrate Polymers. 2019;**203**:310-321

[83] Montero-Lobato Z, Vázquez M, Navarro F, Fuentes JL, Bermejo E, Garbayo I, et al. Chemically-Induced Production of Anti-Inflammatory Molecules in Microalgae. Marine Drugs. 2018;**16**:478

[84] Tabarzad M, Atabaki V, Hosseinabadi T. Anti-inflammatory Activity of Bioactive Compounds from Microalgae and Cyanobacteria by Focusing on the Mechanisms of Action. Molecular Biology Reports. 2020;**47**:6193-6205

[85] Kim S-Y, Roy VC, Park J-S, Chun B-S. Extraction and characterization of bioactive compounds from brown seaweed (Undaria pinnatifida) sporophyll using two sequential green extraction techniques. Algal Research. 2024;**77**:103330

[86] Bojorges H, López-Rubio A, Martínez-Abad A, Fabra MJ. Functional and bioactive properties of the protein-polysaccharide extracts from brown algae: Exploring novel functional ingredients. Food Hydrocolloids. 2025;**162**:110967

[87] Li Y, Qin G, Cheng C, Yuan B, Huang D, Cheng S, et al. Purification, characterization and anti-tumor activities of polysaccharides from Ecklonia kurome obtained by three different extraction methods. International Journal of Biological Macromolecules. 2020;**150**:1000-1010

[88] Suganya AM, Sanjivkumar M, Chandran MN, Palavesam A, Immanuel G. Pharmacological importance of sulphated polysaccharide carrageenan from red seaweed Kappaphycus alvarezii in comparison with commercial carrageenan. Biomedicine and Pharmacotherapy. 2016;**84**:1300-1312

[89] Usoltseva (Menshova) R V, Anastyuk SD, Shevchenko NM, Zvyagintseva TN, Ermakova SP. The comparison of structure and anticancer activity in vitro of polysaccharides from brown algae Alaria marginata and A. angusta. Carbohydrate Polymers. 2016;**153**:258-265

[90] Su F, Song Q, Zhang C, et al. A β-1,3/1,6-glucan from Durvillaea Antarctica inhibits tumor progression in vivo as an immune stimulator. Carbohydrate Polymers. 2019;**222**:114993

[91] Thanh TTT, Quach TMT, Nguyen TN, Vu Luong D, Bui ML, Van TTT. Structure and cytotoxic activity of ulvan extracted from green seaweed Ulva lactuca. International Journal of Biological Macromolecules. 2016;**93**:695-702

[92] Choi JW, Lee J, Kim SC, You S, Lee CW, Shin J, et al. Glucuronorhamnoxylan from Capsosiphon fulvescens inhibits the growth of HT-29 human colon cancer cells in vitro and in vivo via induction of apoptotic cell death. International Journal of Biological Macromolecules. 2019;**124**:1060-1068

[93] Ostad S, Khanavi M, Gheidarloo R, Sadati N, Ardekani MR, Nabavi SB, et al.

Cytotoxicity of fucosterol containing fraction of marine algae against breast and colon carcinoma cell line. Pharmacognosy Magazine. 2012;**8**:60

[94] Luesch H. New apratoxins of marine cyanobacterial origin from guam and palau. Bioorganic & Medicinal Chemistry. 2002;**10**:1973-1978

[95] Catassi A, Cesario A, Arzani D, Menichini P, Alama A, Bruzzo C, et al. Characterization of apoptosis induced by marine natural products in non small cell lung cancer A549 cells. Cellular and Molecular Life Sciences. 2006;**63**:2377-2386

[96] Foster BJ, Fortuna M, Media J, Wiegand RA, Valeriote FA. Cryptophycin 1 cellular levels and effects in vitro using L1210 cells. Investigational New Drugs. 1998;**16**:199-204

[97] Williams DE, Sturgeon CM, Roberge M, Andersen RJ. Nigricanosides A and B, Antimitotic Glycolipids Isolated from the Green Alga *Avrainvillea nigricans* Collected in Dominica. Journal of the American Chemical Society. 2007;**129**:5822-5823

[98] Lee C, Lim K, Kim SS, Thien LX, Lee ES, Oh KT, et al. Chlorella-gold nanorods hydrogels generating photosynthesis-derived oxygen and mild heat for the treatment of hypoxic breast cancer. Journal of Controlled Release. 2019;**294**:77-90

[99] Zhong D, Li W, Hua S, Qi Y, Xie T, Qiao Y, et al. Calcium phosphate engineered photosynthetic microalgae to combat hypoxic-tumor by *in-situ* modulating hypoxia and cascade radio-phototherapy. Theranostics. 2021;**11**:3580-3594

[100] Wang H, Guo Y, Wang C, Jiang X, Liu H, Yuan A, et al. Light-controlled oxygen production and collection for sustainable photodynamic therapy in tumor hypoxia. Biomaterials. 2021;**269**:120621

[101] Zhong D, Zhang D, Chen W, He J, Ren C, Zhang X, et al. Orally deliverable strategy based on microalgal biomass for intestinal disease treatment. Science Advances. 2021;7(48). DOI: 10.1126/sciadv.abi9265

[102] Sekar S, Chandramohan M. Phycobiliproteins as a commodity: trends in applied research, patents and commercialization. Journal of Applied Phycology. 2008;**20**:113-136

[103] Gerber P, Dutcher JD, Adams EV, Sherman JH. Protective Effect of Seaweed Extracts for Chicken Embryos Infected with Influenza B or Mumps Virus. Experimental Biology and Medicine. 1958;**99**:590-593

[104] Besednova NN, Zvyagintseva TN, Kuznetsova TA, Makarenkova ID, Smolina TP, Fedyanina LN, et al. Marine Algae Metabolites as Promising Therapeutics for the Prevention and Treatment of HIV/AIDS. Metabolites. 2019;**9**:87

[105] Kanekiyo K, Hayashi K, Takenaka H, Lee J-B, Hayashi T. Anti-herpes Simplex Virus Target of an Acidic Polysaccharide, Nostoflan, from the Edible Blue-Green Alga Nostoc flagelliforme. Biological & Pharmaceutical Bulletin. 2007;**30**:1573-1575

[106] Wang W, Wang S-X, Guan H-S. The Antiviral Activities and Mechanisms of Marine Polysaccharides: An Overview. Marine Drugs. 2012;**10**:2795-2816

[107] Alam MA, Parra-Saldivar R, Bilal M, Afroze CA, Ahmed MN, Iqbal HMN, et al. Algae-Derived Bioactive Molecules

for the Potential Treatment of SARS-CoV-2. Molecules. 2021;**26**:2134

[108] Sami N, Ahmad R, Fatma T. Exploring algae and cyanobacteria as a promising natural source of antiviral drug against SARS-CoV-2. Biomedical Journal. 2021;**44**:54-62

[109] Salvador N, Garreta AG, Lavelli L, Ribera MA. Antimicrobial activity of Iberian macroalgae. Scientia Marina. 2007;**71**:101-114

[110] Ebrahimi-Mameghani M, Sadeghi Z, Abbasalizad Farhangi M, Vaghef-Mehrabany E, Aliashrafi S. Glucose homeostasis, insulin resistance and inflammatory biomarkers in patients with non-alcoholic fatty liver disease: Beneficial effects of supplementation with microalgae Chlorella vulgaris : A double-blind placebo-controlled randomized clinical trial. Clinical Nutrition. 2017;**36**:1001-1006

[111] Tejani VN, Dhillon SS, Damarlapally N, Usman NUB, Winson T, Basu Roy P, et al. The Relationship Between Dietary Fiber Intake and Blood Pressure Worldwide: A Systematic Review. Cureus. 2023;**15**(9):e46116. DOI: 10.7759/cureus.46116

[112] Minhas LA, Kaleem M, Farooqi HMU, Kausar F, Waqar R, Bhatti T, et al. Algae-derived bioactive compounds as potential pharmaceuticals for cancer therapy: A comprehensive review. Algal Research. 2024;**78**:103396

[113] Yao W, Qiu H-M, Cheong K-L, Zhong S. Advances in anti-cancer effects and underlying mechanisms of marine algae polysaccharides. International Journal of Biological Macromolecules. 2022;**221**:472-485

[114] Hannan MA, Sohag AAM, Dash R, Haque MN, Mohibbullah M, Oktaviani DF, et al. Phytosterols of marine algae: Insights into the potential health benefits and molecular pharmacology. Phytomedicine. 2020;**69**:153201

[115] Zhou J, Wang M, Pallarés N, Ferrer E, Berrada H, Barba FJ. Sterols and fat-soluble vitamins. In: Food Lipids. Netherlands: Elsevier; 2022. pp. 323-348

[116] Mao Z, Shen X, Dong P, Liu G, Pan S, Sun X, et al. Fucosterol exerts antiproliferative effects on human lung cancer cells by inducing apoptosis, cell cycle arrest and targeting of Raf/MEK/ERK signalling pathway. Phytomedicine. 2019;**61**:152809

[117] Raman M, Doble M. κ-Carrageenan from marine red algae, Kappaphycus alvarezii – A functional food to prevent colon carcinogenesis. Journal of Functional Foods. 2015;**15**:354-364

[118] Han D, Zhang X, Ma Y, Yang X, Li Z. The development of live microorganism-based oxygen shuttles for enhanced hypoxic tumor therapy. Materials Today Bio. 2023;**18**:100517

[119] Xin Z, Zhang M, Cui H, Ding X, Zhang T, Wu L, et al. Algae: A Robust Living Material Against Cancer. International Journal of Nanomedicine. 2023;**18**:5243-5264

[120] Zhong D, Li W, Qi Y, He J, Zhou M. Photosynthetic Biohybrid Nanoswimmers System to Alleviate Tumor Hypoxia for FL/PA/MR Imaging-Guided Enhanced Radio-Photodynamic Synergetic Therapy. Advanced Functional Materials. 2020;**30**(17). DOI: 10.1002/adfm.201910395

[121] de la Asunción-Nadal V, Franco C, Veciana A, et al. MoSBOTs: Magnetically Driven Biotemplated $MoS_2$-Based

Microrobots for Biomedical Applications. Small. 2022;**18**(33):2203821. DOI: 10.1002/smll.202203821

[122] Dagnino-Leone J, Figueroa CP, Castañeda ML, Youlton AD, Vallejos-Almirall A, Agurto-Muñoz A, et al. Phycobiliproteins: Structural aspects, functional characteristics, and biotechnological perspectives. Computational and Structural Biotechnology Journal. 2022;**20**:1506-1527

[123] Kronick MN. The use of phycobiliproteins as fluorescent labels in immunoassay. Journal of Immunological Methods. 1986;**92**:1-13

[124] Future Market Insights Inc. Global Phycocyanin Market Snapshot (2023 to 2033); 2023. Available from: https://www.futuremarketinsights.com/reports/phycocyanin-market [Accessed: December 30, 2024]

Chapter 3

# Bio-Mitigation of Carbon Dioxide Using Microalgae Cultivated in Tubular-Photobioreactor

*Ahmed Aidan Al-Hussieny*


## Abstract

Bio-mitigation lowers greenhouse gas technology dioxide levels. *Chlorella sorokiniana* during a 24-day laboratory study period were evaluated at five distinct $CO_2$ concentrations: 5, 10, 15, 20, and 25 L/min while being cultivated in nitrogen, phosphorus, and potassium (NPK) growth media. The $CO_2$ removal rate employed was 92.94% including proteins, lipids, phenols, flavones, glycosyrosiates, anthocyanins, and carotenoids, whereas the greatest level of gas was 25 L/min or 6000 mg/L. The biomass's greatest proportion of proteins and lipids for the highest rate of gas (25 L/min) reached 47.08%, respectively, and 34.05% relative to the control 31.32% and 20.35%, respectively, as measured by its 0.102 nm difference from the control, and through the efficiency of the isolate of Chl. *sorokiniana*. It was tested by reducing the highest $CO_2$ levels of 25 L/min within a 200 L photo bioreactor design. with a period of 24 days in the laboratory's natural environment. After harvesting the algal reactor cultivation of 200 L, the biomass weight reached 900 g/L. This means that for every 1 g of algae biomass, 1.7 g of $CO_2$ is consumed.


**Keywords:** protein, carbon dioxide, nitrogen phosphate potassium (NPK), algae, culture

## 1. Introduction

One of the major issues that humanity has faced throughout its long history is climate change, which has a direct impact on the climate of the planet and, in turn, on people and other living things. Since the middle of the nineteenth century, human activities, including the burning of fossil fuels, have led to high atmospheric concentrations of greenhouse gases (GHGs) and the average temperature rising of the earth's surface. Extreme weather, ozone depletion, increased risk of wildfires, loss of biodiversity, stress on food production systems, the global spread of infectious diseases, and economic and social implications are only a few of the negative aspects of climate change that are directly tied to human health [1], Therefore, the world gets warmer as a result of emissions of greenhouse gases from businesses and human activity. According to the Fourth Assessment Report of the Intergovernmental Panel on Climate Change (IPCC), published in 2007, an increase in emissions might result in a temperature increase of 4–7°C, having a significant impact on the environment and human activity [2].

For many years, the main factor driving companies that emit $CO_2$ is to blame for the rise in greenhouse gases in the environment. Hence, using fossil fuels for home use, transportation, electricity, and heat is the main cause of greenhouse gas emissions worldwide. Certain forms of algae, during their exponential growth, can double the biomass in short periods of time of up to 3.5 hours. This is because capture and storage, in particular, is currently a serious technological and global concern. Algae are highly effective at eliminating and tolerating high carbon dioxide concentrations [3]. Algae consume large amounts of carbon dioxide through photosynthesis and convert it as a food source. In addition, the algae contribute nearly 40–50% of the oxygen in the atmosphere, thereby helping to support the majority of life on our planet [4]. They are very effective feedstock for biodiesel production [5]. mentioned that some algal species have been found to have very high oil contents, ranging up to and sometimes beyond 50% of dry weight. Algae-based carbon dioxide ($CO_2$) sequestration has drawn increased attention since it can use $CO_2$ as a source of carbon. Stronger growth rates than typical crop plants, improved culture conditions, and increased photosynthetic efficiency and $CO_2$ fixation capacity. The generated biomass can be utilized as a feedstock for a variety of products with added value, such as ethanol and chemicals [6]. The ability of microalgae to be a workable $CO_2$ sequestration technology has attracted modern attention in its development. This form of gas can be gathered and turned into energy sources [3, 7, 8].

## 2. Study objective

- Bio-mitigation for the concentration of $CO_2$ using different species of coccoid green algae in a photobioreactor (PBRs) and producing biomass from algae.

- Evaluating the effectiveness of these species in the mitigation of biological $CO_2$ processes.

- The utilization of algal biomass in various applications, including the production of lipids as a source of biofuels as well as proteins.

## 3. Global warming

Global warming is a serious environmental problem. This is typically blamed for an increase in the atmospheric concentration of greenhouse gases (GHGs), particularly ($CO_2$) carbon dioxide [9], as well as methane, tropospheric ozone, and chlorofluorocarbons. It is a factor in the steady warming of Earth's climatic system that has been seen since the pre-industrial era (between 1850 and 1900), mostly as a result of fossil fuel use by humans increasing the levels of greenhouse gases that trap heat in the Earth's atmosphere [10].

Carbon dioxide is considered a hazardous gas in the atmosphere as it is mainly responsible for changing (60–63%) of different layers of the atmosphere from 1979 to 2004 [11].

So anthropogenic carbon dioxide ($CO_2$) emissions, which are now largely from fossil fuel combustion and also from terrestrial carbon stocks from land use change, have increased the atmospheric $CO_2$ concentration [9]. Excessive radiative forcing from rising emissions of carbon dioxide and other greenhouse gases (GHGs) is already disrupting the climate in many ways. Damage includes ice cover and glaciers, sea level rise, extreme weather, ocean acidification, greater variability in agricultural and forest production, including risks of crop failure, damage to ecosystems, spread of disease, and other risks to humans and other life forms [12].

Familiar alternative renewable energy technologies and methods, such as solar, wind, ocean, geothermal, bioethanol, biodiesel, wood, or hydrogen have potential for recycling and low pollution impacts [13].

For that, global biofuel markets have grown quickly over the last five years, indicating renewed interest in these fuels. However, what is novel about this renewed interest and what makes biofuels a serious option for partially replacing oil as a transportation fuel are their alleged lower greenhouse gas (GHG) emissions. This would make it easier for nations to fight the issue of global warming and fulfill their obligations under the Kyoto Protocol. Additionally, the Brazilian experience demonstrates that biofuels can promote rural development and export potential. This would make it easier for nations to fight the issue of global warming and fulfill their obligations under the Kyoto Protocol. Additionally, the Brazilian experience demonstrates that biofuels can promote rural development and export potential [14].

Although petroleum and coal have been the primary energy sources used for a long time due to their high abundance, high energy content, and low pricing, biofuels have been available for a long time. While fossil fuels like coal and petroleum also originate from biomass, their production requires millions of years. Due to rising oil prices, depleting fossil fuel reserves, the need for a dependable, renewable energy source, and a strategy to lessen the consequences of climate change, biofuels are experiencing a renaissance. Because they are constantly renewed, biofuels are renewable resources. On the other hand, because they take millions of years to produce, fossil fuels cannot be renewed.

Biofuels come from modern living organisms over a short period of time, differing from fossil fuels also in the same way, through the decomposition of organic matter, but over many years [15]. In addition, biofuels do not lead to acid rain and have few adverse effects on the environment because they contain less sulfur and reduce carbon dioxide emissions [14].

## 4. Algae as a biofuel source

Microalga oil is now thought of as a possible biodiesel feedstock alternative. The production of biofuels now requires significantly more oil than is available; hence, it is necessary to employ alternative biomass sources. Microalgae outperform land-based plants in a variety of ways when it comes to producing oil. They may generate more oil per spot than high-quality oilseed crops, thanks to their simple unicellular structure and strong photosynthetic efficiency. Algae can form at the interface with brackish or salt water, which means they no longer compete with traditional agriculture for resources. They should be grown in conjunction with the absorption of $CO_2$ from industrial waste streams, removal of excess nutrients from wastewater, and the discontinuance of the use of herbicides and pesticides [16].

In addition to oil production, it is needed to produce by-products such as pigments, antioxidants, nutritional supplements, fertilizers, and animal feed [17]. Despite these benefits, algal gas is currently not widely used, typically because of its high production costs [5, 18]. Despite strong economic interest from industry and researchers, there are currently no commercial plants producing biodiesel from algae [19]. The production of biomass and lipids by the algae is one of the major technological and economical barriers in the system [20].

A productive strain and ideal living conditions are required to produce cells with a high growth rate, and at the same time, a high fat content. The high cost and energy requirements for harvesting unicellular algae are another significant challenge. The small cell size (typically 10 m in diameter) and the dilute biomass produced require new strategies to reduce the amount of water and energy consumed, as well as processing costs [21].

## 5. Classification of microalgae

Microalgae are tiny organisms that perform photosynthesis by absorbing sunlight and transforming it into chemical energy. Their diameter varies between 1 and 30 μm [22]. They are diverse groups of organisms, do not contain leaves, stems, and roots, and consist of chlorophyll to follow the process of photosynthesis [11] and microalgae can be classified into prokaryotic, eukaryotic, heterotrophic, autotrophic, mixotrophic, non-photosynthetic, and photosynthetic [23].

Microalgal organisms reach in size from unicellular (microalgae) to multicellular (macroalgae) and grow in the aquatic environment [23]. Macroalgae was not very effective in the development of experimental biofuel compared to microalgae—the structure is more complex, has a slower growth rate, and has less oil content [24].

The fewer properties of macroalgae compared to microalgae lead to some limitations in terms of macroalgae in biofuel production [24]. However, the microalgae harvesting process is more complicated than macroalgae [25]. Microalgae can be phototrophic (the energy source being light during photosynthesis) as well as heterotrophic (cells require only carbon as an energy source) [26]. Microalgae are photosynthetic, and they perform photosynthesis using carbon dioxide and sunlight to produce organic formulations to promote their growth.

There are about 50,000 different types of microalgae, but only a few of them have been described [23]. The main divisions of microalgae in terms of their pigmentation are green, blue-green, brown, red, and gold microalgae [27].

Among the microalgae that are distinguished in the Iraqi aquatic environment inside the Euphrates River are *Rhabdoderma hamiformi* and *Komvophoron schmidlei*, belonging to the blue-green microalgae [28]. *Chlorella sorokiniana* and *Coelastrella* sp. belong to green microalgae that are employed in the present study and recognized in the Iraq environment (Tigris River) by [29].

## 6. Advantages of microalgae for biofuel production

The scarcity of petrochemical resources and environmental contamination are two pressing issues that our civilization needs to address. Petroleum oil shortages and the rise in gasoline prices are now significant issues in limiting the global economy due to the world's finite supply of petroleum and its ongoing depletion. Also, the results of scientific literature indicate that the massive usage of fossil fuels, which results in global warming and climate-related disasters, is the primary source of environmental contamination. Both social and industrial researchers are now seeking renewable energy alternatives that can partially replace fossil fuel resources to develop a more sustainable society and encourage global economic recovery in order to address these issues. One example of renewable energy that comes from biomass is [30]. In addition to addressing the issue of energy scarcity, biomass energy is significantly more environmentally friendly than fossil fuel. Terrestrial crops, the first- and second-generation feed stocks for biofuels, present new difficulties, such as the encroachment of arable land, which results in a food crisis [31].

Macroalgae and microalgae are the two basic categories of algae. Brown algae, red algae, and green seaweed are examples of macroalgae. Green algae, Spirulina, and Chlorella are examples of microalgae. The marine and freshwater environments are home to more than 20,000 different types of microalgae. Unfortunately, so far, only a few types of microalgae have been discovered that can convert biomass into energy. Microalgae offers more advantages than macroalgae, including simple structures, rapid development, high oil content, and other factors. As a result, the majority of industrial businesses prefer to employ microalgae as the raw materials for biomass energy production [32].

## 7. The role of carbon dioxide in increasing the mass of microalgae

Microalgae are mostly found near or in water bodies, and they are necessary for both terrestrial and aquatic habitats. Algae species number over 70,000, yet the majority of them are unsuitable for human consumption. Algae can be raised in environments that are not ideal for the growth of common crops like soybeans and others. Algae have the potential to fix $CO_2$ in the climate and help reduce the expansion of carbon dioxide levels in the air, which is an important global issue [11].

So it is considered Carbon (C), the most crucial component for microalgal growth, followed by nitrogen (N) and phosphorus (P) (microalgal biomass contains around 50% carbon, all of which is produced from $CO_2$). Because the creation of 1 g of microalgal biomass yields about 1.83 g of $CO_2$ fixation, these microorganisms can be used to successfully fix $CO_2$ [33]. Microalgae can fix $CO_2$ from both the atmosphere and flue gas emissions. When choosing a location for the microalgal facility, using atmospheric $CO_2$ gives you more freedom because you do not need to put it near a source of $CO_2$ emissions and you do not need $CO_2$ transporting equipment [34]. Several studies have reported the use of microalgae in $CO_2$ capture from the atmosphere [35]. Only a few studies have reported the use of real flue gases for microalgal growth. When growing *Chlorella* sp. in an outdoor open thin layer PBR using a flue gas containing 6–8% of $CO_2$, reported $CO_2$ removal efficiencies between 10 and 50% [36] when cultivating *Scenedesmus* flue gas obliquus with a content of 6–18%. The best species to collect from these gaseous streams are native species that are isolated from thermal power facilities, according to some experts.

## 8. Possible applications for the biomass of microalgae

It costs money to cultivate microalgae for $CO_2$ absorption. But if the biomass generated serves other uses in addition to reducing carbon emissions, it can be made commercially viable. Algae biomass may be crucial in ensuring the security of both animal and human food supplies. Because they contain a variety of vital elements, including vitamins, minerals, and polyunsaturated fatty acids, microalgae have a high nutritional value [37]. *Chlorella, Spirulina, Scenedesmus*, and *Caelastrum* sp. have a protein level of 60%, while these microalgae include 18 of the 22 recognized amino acids [38]. They include sulfur-containing essential amino acids that are typically absent from most human diets [39]. They also include a significant amount of polyunsaturated fatty acids, such as arachidonic acid, docosahexaenoic acid, hexadecatrienoic acid, octadecatetraenoic acid, omega 3 fatty acids, and hexadecatetraenoic acid methyl ester [40]. Fish bred in aquaculture hatcheries as well as other animals are all thought to benefit from eating microalgae as a healthy source of protein. However, microalgae grown in sewage treatment plant effluents should not be consumed by humans, animals, or fish as they can contain many contaminants such as pathogens, viruses, heavy metals, and pesticide residues. Microalgae also comprise bioactive substances that are useful for medicinal purposes [41]. Algae are a good source of nutraceuticals due to a number of them, including sterols, toxins, and lipid antioxidants like carotene [42]. Humans are thought to benefit from consuming microalgae, a high-protein food source. Microalgae-based therapeutic effect therapies on ailments associated with oxidative stress have drawn a lot of attention [43]. Microalgae have properties that make them useful for treating a range of medical conditions. They inhibit swelling, convulsions, and inflammation in addition to acting as analgesics, bronchodilators, antibacterial, and polysynaptic blockers, among other things. Algal biomass has substances It may be used to create income for industries. Moreover, microalgae create oils, pigments, polysaccharides, dyes, and bio-flocculants [44]. Phycobiliproteins are fluorescent dyes employed in specific immunoassays and cell separations. Other advantageous substances include astaxanthin, lutein, zeaxanthin, lycopene, and bixin [43, 45].

## 9. Types of photobioreactors (PBRs)

### 9.1 Serpentine photobioreactors

They consist of a flat loop (the photo stage) formed from straight tubes connected at U-bends that can be positioned either vertically or horizontally. A pump or an airlift is used to achieve in a separate vessel, gas exchange and nutrient input frequently occur, while culture circulation (at flow rates between 20 and 30 cm s) occurs simultaneously [46] designed a tube-shaped photo bioreactor to grow *Arthrospira*. It was made of flexible polyethylene sleeves with a thickness of and a diameter of 14 cm 0.3 mm that were joined together to form a loop using polyvinyl chloride (PVC) bends, each of which had a tiny oxygen-releasing tube The pilot plant had two distinct components (500 m long, 8 $m^3$ in volume, and 80 $m^2$ in surface area). Portphyridium was produced in a similar tubular photo bioreactor. The loop was constructed using polyethylene [46] tubes with 6.4 cm diameter and 1500 m length. The top layer was either floated or submerged on top of or in a pool filled with people to control the temperature of the manner of life as shown in **Figure 1**.

### 9.2 Manifold photobioreactors

In manifold PBRs, there are two manifolds: one is used for distribution, and the other is used for repeating the same suspension in series are used to connect a group of parallel tubes at their ends. Due to the suspended float distance between the tube inlet and the degasser and the reduced oxygen concentrations, these structures have two key advantages over serpentine loop PBRs that make to an industrial scale level easier [46]. Created a system for the first time that consisted of manifold-connected parallel sets of 20-m-long tubes that allowed airlifts to circulate the culture. With

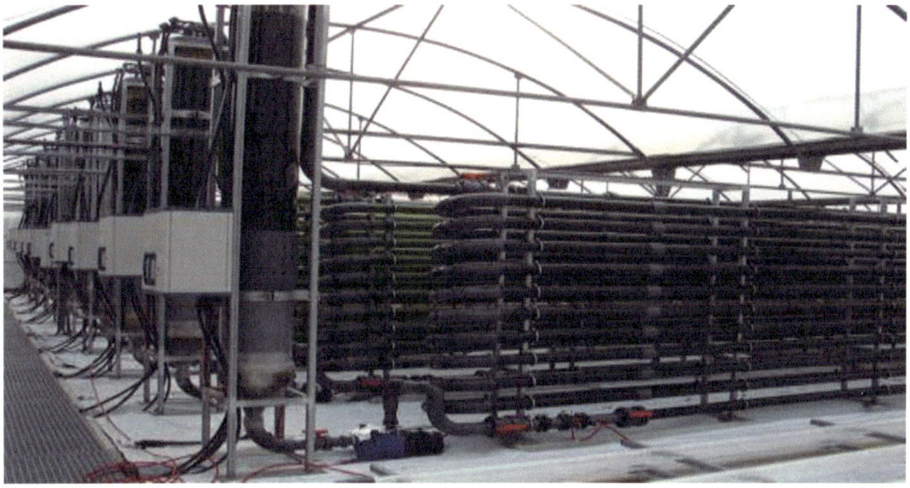

**Figure 1.**
*The University of Almeria's department of chemical engineering created a vertical tubular serpentine photo bioreactor (Spain) [47].*

*Arthospira* sp., productivity levels of 0.55 g were obtained. The Near-Horizontal Tubular Reactor (NHTR), created by [46], has tubes with an angle of 5–20° (**Figure 2**).

### 9.3 Helical photobioreactors

PBR helices are composed of tubes that can bend with a tiny inner diameter looped around an upright supporting framework. The development of *Chlorella* sp. used this design in the 1950s, and it was later adopted by [43]. Formerly, *Anabaena platensis* and *Anabaena siamensis* were grown outside in a 120-l helical bubble PBR. For A. *platensis*, a PE of 6.6%for photosynthetic activity (PAR) and an implied volumetric productiveness of 0.9 g l d 1 have been achieved [46]. A bio coil made of a photo stage of 2.5–5 cm diameter polyethylene or PVC tubing that has been helically wound around a cylindrical structure that is 8 m high and has a 2 m core diameter. The pumping system has connected many parallel bands of tubes using manifolds, enabling more uniform gliding and shorter tube lengths to prevent oxygen accumulation [46]. Temperature control was provided by a warming trade or evaporative cooling. In Perth, Western Australia, the cyanobacterium *Arthrospira* sp. and other marine species have been raised in a 1000-l Bio coil [39]. Unfortunately, there has been little recent discussion of the Bio coil shows that it is no longer in use. Very useful. Moreover, a conical framework has been proposed as opposed to a cylindrical one because it enhances the geographical provision of tubes to daylight seize [46]. Small conical biocoil devices operate now and in the past in most cases for test purposes and educating functions [35].

### 9.4 Tubular PBRs for special applications

Condensed photovoltaic radiation-using tubular serpentine PBR has been installed in the Nové Hrady Academic and University Center [48]. The PBR is entirely

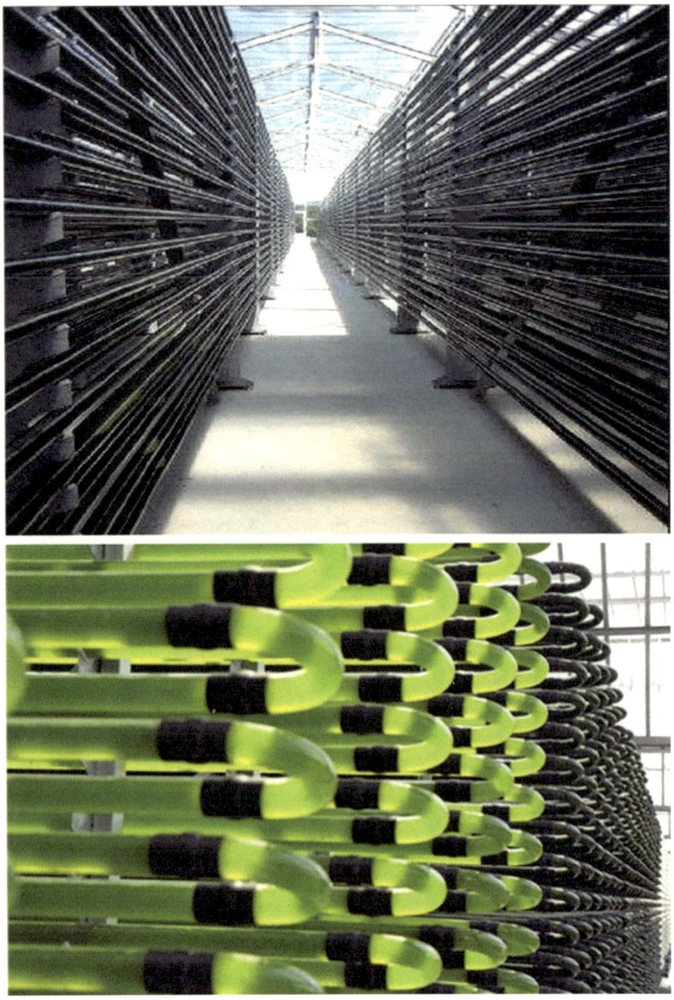

**Figure 2.**
*Installed photobioreactors with a tubular manifold by Roquette Klötze & Co. (Germany) has tubular manifold photobioreactors installed.*

supported by photovoltaic concentrators installed in a greenhouse with climate control, which concentrate the cultivation tubes' direct exposure to sunlight as it falls. The farming component is mounted on a movable frame that enables computerized concentrating of direct photovoltaic irradiation. The 24-m-long cultivation unit is a U-shaped loop constructed of six horizontals, parallel glass tubes. With irradiance values as high as 3.5 times what is naturally feasible, the PBR has been used to investigate how microalgae adapt to supra-high photovoltaic irradiation [48]. Depending on an upgraded, two-stage (PBR) with two vertical, and there were two inclined units created and examined based on this initial design, as illustrated in **Figure 3** [49].

It is possible to produce biomass in two stages using the innovative 450-l PBR: I by growing the chosen microalga at both I by exposing the culture to excessively the tilted units have a high irradiance and (ii) by using lower irradiances in the vertical units. The red phase in the inclined units and the green phase in the vertical units of this method have both been evaluated for the generation of *H. pluvialis* [49]. The

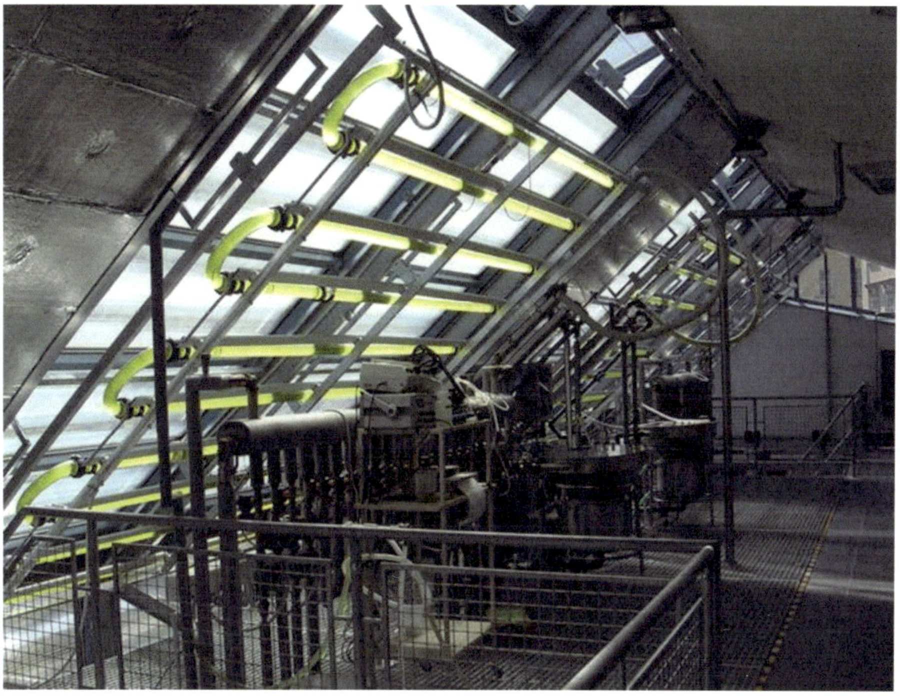

**Figure 3.**
*A linear Fresnel lens-based solar concentrator-based tubular serpentine photo bioreactor was created at the University of South Bohemia's center for biotechnology in Nové Hrady (Czech Republic).*

technique makes it possible to grow microalgae at irradiances that are significantly higher than those that are natural, which might be advantageous at high latitudes. Also, it subjects the culture to the extremely high irradiances needed to stress organisms and collect valuable compounds (Colors, Superoxide Dismutase, etc.). The key technological limitation is the PBR's high price, which is approximately €1000 and includes glass tubes, Fresnel lenses, a light tracking system, a degasser, a heat exchanger, a pump, sensors, and a control box [48]. To circumvent the problem of light saturation effect, which is actually a great drawback in microalgal biotechnology [46], have recently proposed a new tubular PBR design in which the culture tubes are arranged on an 8 × 8 square pitch cell connected by U-bends and immersed in a light-scattering silica nanoparticle suspension.

## 10. Design algal tubular photobioreactor

The working mechanism featured a tubular photo bioreactor that receives 25 L/min of $CO_2$ gas through a down-of-the-ground conveyor tube that is supported by the other vertical tubes. The process of accurately stirring the culture media containing algae was made possible by the appearance of gas with minute bubbles filled with algae cells following agricultural medium NPK propagation in the presence of outside natural conditions as an applied work 100% in winter, along with a drop in temperature and lighting intensity. An air pump is installed on the upper conveyor to help the algae move toward the culture tank. In addition, a monitor is in charge of the higher conveyor. When

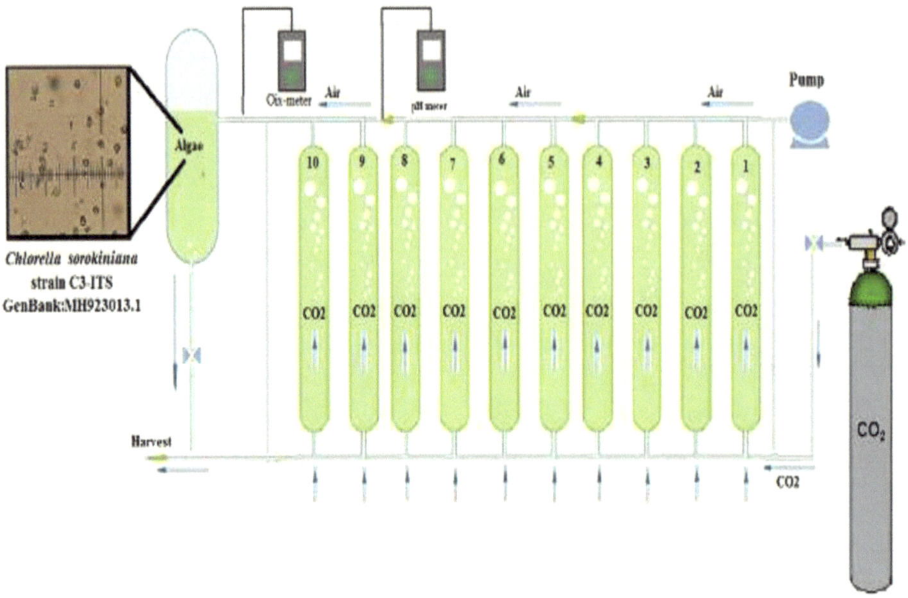


**Figure 4.**
Chlorella sorokiniana *is used to illustrate the algae photo bioreactor (PBRs) mechanism for the biological reduction of* $CO_2$.

introducing the algal flow into the growth tank, use a pH-meter and an OIX-meter equipment to determine the pH levels and initial yield of dissolved oxygen, respectively. There is a tap for the algal harvesting process to collect the biomass at the bottom of the culture tank, and there are two 10-liter reactors for each reactor as a control or point of comparison for the algal reactor. $CO_2$ gas is installed in the first reactor at the same level as the reactor (25 L/min.) in comparison to reducing the gas, and the second reactor, which simply supplies air and does not utilize $CO_2$ gas, is outfitted with an air pump. Whereas, the algal bioreactor's carrying capacity was 200 L of the algae cultures that were used to reduce the gas, and **Figure 4** shows the shape of the algal bioreactor.

## 11. $CO_2$ reduction by *Chlorella sorokiniana* in an algal reactor

Micro-green algae have high efficiency in the process of absorbing nutrients from the environment through a specialized enzyme mechanism in the cell wall. In addition to its size, it gave it coverage of wide surface areas, especially in closed algal reactor systems equipped with a carbon source in the form of $CO_2$ gas. The gas concentrations were measured in mg /L unit by using a gas measuring device ($CO_2$) before preparing the bioreactor and the first control with $CO_2$ gas. It was found that the gas in the bioreactor has a concentration of 991 mg/L, and they are a result of an air pump in the reactor. In the first control reactor, the concentration of $CO_2$ gas reached 522 mg/L, also due to the air pump that works to dissolve the gas as it is pure gas, and the second control reactor reached 327 mg/L, also due to the air pump. After the bioreactor and the first control reactor were equipped with gas in an amount of 25 L/min, which corresponds to 6000 mg/L and after 24 hours from the start of the experiment, the gas concentration in the algae reactor reached 1460 mg/L with a removal rate of 75.6%, which is the result of the exponential increase in the light density of algae. After 48 hours, the gas reached 38 mg/L with a removal rate of 99.3%, and after 72 hours, the gas reached 10 mg/L, with a removal rate of 99.8%. Compared to the first control, in which the gas mechanism after 24 hours reached 4600 mg/L, with a removal rate of 23.3%, and after 48 hours it reached 2750 mg/L, and a removal rate of 54.1%, and after 72 hours, the gas reached 1689 mg/L with a removal rate of 71.8%.

## 12. Biochemical examinations

### 12.1 Protein

After the experiment was completed, the algal cultures were harvested (in the algal reactor and the first and second control cultures) the wet mass was converted to dry and chemical and biological analyses were conducted. Among the analyses, there were different percentages of protein between the algae reactor equipped with a $CO_2$ gas rate of 25 L/min, the first control equipped with gas and the second control without gas processing. The results showed the protein percentages to 50.1, 27.2, and 21.4%, respectively, as presented in **Table 1**.

### 12.2 Lipid

One of the most promising approaches to reducing carbon dioxide emissions from the energy sector is biological carbon dioxide fixation, particularly through the deployment of technically sound photosynthesis systems. According to studies, the method can be used to reduce carbon dioxide through the process of photosynthesis by using microalgae, both in terms of cost and environmental impact. Being a modern and environmentally friendly technology for biological carbon sequestration in algae culture and the production of biomass for cultured algae, it is 10–20 times more effective than the technology employed in other plants in reducing and seizing this gas emitted to the gas envelope. The added value of the algae biomass produced after the bio-building process is used as a result of taking advantage of the $CO_2$ gas, whereby the algae biomass can be used in various applications, including the production of fats as a source of biofuels. In the current research, the percentage of lipids within algae biomass was 33.2, 21.3, and 17.2%, respectively (**Table 2**).

### 12.3 Carbohydrate

Carbohydrates constitute a small part of the cell components in microalgae, but they contribute significantly to their nutritional value. The percentage of

| Name | Protein % | Lipid % | Total carbohydrate % | TPC mg gallic /gm | TFC mg rutin /gm |
|---|---|---|---|---|---|
| Tubular photobioreactor (PBRs) | 50.1 | 33.2 | 13.2 | 27.8 | 19.2 |
| Control with $CO_2$ | 27.2 | 21.3 | 9.7 | 14.4 | 11.8 |
| Control without $CO_2$ | 21.4 | 17.2 | 4.6 | 12.1 | 9.24 |

**Table 1.**
Chlorella sorokiniana *biomass was processed for its biochemical components, which were then cultivated in a tubular photobioreactor with pure $CO_2$ gas.*

| Name reactor | TGC % | *T. antho* (ppm) | *T. carotene* (ppm) |
|---|---|---|---|
| Tubular photo bioreactor (PBRs) | 3.01 | 2.33 | 16.48 |
| Control with $CO_2$ | 2.23 | 1.05 | 10.12 |
| Control without $CO_2$ | 1.45 | 0.95 | 6.65 |

**Table 2.**
*Chemical mixtures extracted in a tubular photobioreactor at a rate of 25 L/min from the biomass of the algae* Chlorella sorokiniana.

carbohydrates in the current study within the algal biomass was 13.2, 9.7, and 4.6%, respectively, and total carbohydrates were the third in the biochemical content of *Chlorella sorokiniana*, compared to the control (**Table 2**).

### 12.4 Total phenolic compounds

The concentrations of phenols within the algal biomass reached 27.8, 14.4, and 12.1 mg Gallic/gm, respectively, for the algal reactor at a $CO_2$ rate of 25 L/min, the first control equipped with gas, and the second control without gas preparation (**Table 2**).

### 12.5 Glycoside

Glycoside is one of the products of *Chlorella sorokiniana* in biomass produced in a culture medium that contains $CO_2$ in a photovoltaic reactor during the study period of 24 days. After harvesting algae biomass, the percentage of glycoside was 3.01, 2.23, and 1.45%, respectively, as shown in **Table 2**.

### 12.6 Anthocyanin

Anthocyanin pigments are secondary metabolites of algae and terrestrial plants that have a major role in plant (algal) cell physiology first by acting as visual signals to animals to aid in inducing pollination and seed dispersal. It depends on increasing its concentrations on the carbon source, as shown by the current research, despite the amount of gas supplied to the algae reactor, which is 25 L/min. The dye concentration reached 2.33 mg/L compared to the control reactors equipped with gas at an intensity of 1.05 mg/L and the $CO_2$-free control of 0.95 mg/L as shown in **Table 2**.

### 12.7 Carotene total

The concentration of carotene pigment within the biomass of *Chlorella sorokiniana* was 16.48, 10.12, and 6.65 mg/L, respectively, as shown in **Table 2**. Algal biomass is of great importance for the size and proportion of biochemical products, including carotenoid pigments.

### 12.8 Fatty acids

Fatty acids are a crucial and influential part of determining the biochemical content, economic and nutritional value of microalgae. It is clear from the present study that the biomass of *Chlorella sorokiniana* contains different types and percentages of fatty acids, including Palmatic (C16:0), Oleic (C18:1), Linoleic (C18:2), Stearic (C18:0), EICOSANOIC (C20), A – Lenolinic (C18:3), Myristate (C14:0), Hexanoate

| Some important fatty acids (%) | Name of reactor | | |
|---|---|---|---|
| | Tubular photobioreactor | Control with $CO_2$ | Control without $CO_2$ |
| Saturated fatty acids | | | |
| Palmatic<br>C16:0 | 12.6 | 9.3 | 5.8 |
| Myristate<br>C:14:0 | 3.86 | 2.06 | 1.032 |
| Hexanoate<br>C6:0 | 8.48 | 4.21 | 2.54 |
| Stearic<br>C18:0 | 5.9 | 3.7 | 1.9 |
| Arachidate<br>C20:0 | 4.12 | 1.65 | 0.92 |
| Unsaturated fatty acids | | | |
| Oleic<br>C18:1 | 20.8 | 12.6 | 9.32 |
| Linoleic<br>C18:2 | 10.9 | 7.5 | 5.8 |
| Eicosanoic<br>C20:0 | 17.5 | 12.8 | 9.8 |
| Docosahexa<br>C22:6 | 7.38 | 3.98 | 1.54 |
| A – Lenolinic<br>C18:3 | 9.8 | 5.43 | 4.6 |

**Table 3.**
*Percentages of saturated and unsaturated fatty acids recovered from* Chlorella sorokiniana *biomass cultivated in a tubular photo bioreactor under 25 L/min of $CO_2$ gas using gas chromatography (GC) techniques.*

(C6:0), Arachidate (C20:0), and Docosahexa (C22:6) with different percentages amounting to 12.6, 20.8, 10.9, 5.9, 17.5, and 9.8%, respectively. For an algal reactor equipped with an amount of 25 L/min of $CO_2$ gas compared to the Control with $CO_2$ 9.3, 12.6, 7.5, 3.7, 12.8, and 6.9%, respectively, and compared the Control without $CO_2$ 5.8, 10.9, 5.8, 1.9, 9.8, and 4.6%, respectively, as presented in **Table 3**.

## 13. Percentage of biological compounds within a culture of *Chlorella sorokiniana*

Due to the reliance of the world's economy on fossil fuels, $CO_2$, the primary gas causing global warming, is responsible for more than half of all other greenhouse gases (GHGs). Due to its unmatched advantages over higher plants, algal biotechnology is the most promising method for biologically sequestering carbon dioxide using microalgae [50]. Construct a closed gas handling system while using an open pond or closed photo bioreactor (PBR) system for autotrophic production. Microalgae had a photosynthetic efficiency of 10–20%, compared to most terrestrial plants' 1–2%.

Biomass of *Chlorella soroquiniana* grown with $CO_2$ gas medium in a PBR included a 50.1% greater amount of protein than the other products. The percentage of lipids was next (33.2%), followed by that of carbs (13.2%), as shown in **Figure 5**.

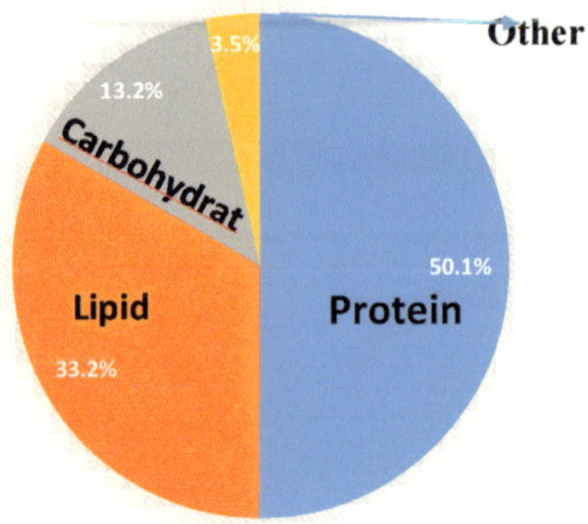


**Figure 5.**
*The chemical chemicals found in* Chlorella sorokiniana *biomass grown in the Tubular-BPR culture and equipped with a rate of 25 L/min. of $CO_2$ gas for 24 days.*

The protein content of algae may reach 50–70% of the dry weight of the algal mass of the phylum blue-green algae. It exceeds the content of meat, eggs, powdered milk, cereals, and soybeans, as well as being a high-quality protein that includes every necessary amino acid, especially leucine, valine, and isoleucine. This shows a high digestibility of 83–90% due to the lack of cellulose walls. Unlike other microorganisms proposed as protein sources, such as algae (*Chlorella* and *Scenedesmus*), which have cellulose walls isolating several antibiotics from algae which showed great chemical diversity [40]. In recent research, it was found that algae-based proteins can block the entry of HIV. Instead of extracting the vaccine; people can eat the algae directly and let their bodies metabolize the pollen [51].

Carbohydrates constitute a small part of the cell components in microalgae, but they play an important role in their nutritional value and the ability to digest the algal mass by the organisms feeding on it. Its cells contain Glucose, Xylose, Mannose, and Galactose, as the content of the alga *Scenedesmus* sp. (from microalgae) of total carbohydrates is about 12.50% of the dry weight and 13.50% of the dry weight of *Chlorella* sp. But it is low in blue-green algae such as *Spirulina* sp. The total carbohydrate content ranges between 8 and 14% of the dry weight. Where the bulk of carbohydrates are discovered is in the green algae cell walls and not found in blue-green algae because they are prokaryotic organisms. As for the lipid content of algal cells, it depends on the algae culture conditions. It was noted that there is a wide variation in its lipid content, which ranges between 2 and 20% of the dry weight and may reach 80% of the dry weight in some algal species, as in *Botryococcus braunii* (a green alga) and under suitable cultivation conditions [5]. The reason for this is due to the extraction method used, for example, the total lipid content of the alga *Spirulina platensis* ranged between 5.6 and 7% of the dry weight and could reach more than that when using better extraction methods [52].

The variation in the proportions of protein, lipids, and carbohydrates within the algal biomass is the result of the different conditions of algae culture and the difference between the culture media and their concentrations. As well as the temperature, pH values, intensity of illumination, and the provision of a carbon source with a high concentration. The study [5] matched the percentages of algal products such as protein, lipid, and carbohydrates to 45.02, 22.89, and 21.11%, respectively, within a culture medium equipped with a high-level carbon source as well as the study [53, 54].

## 14. Conclusions

1. The photo bioreactor proved its efficiency in reducing the highest rate of $CO_2$ gas of 25 L/min, with a reduction rate of 99.3% after 48 hours from the start of the experiment.

2. The total productivity alga *Chlorella sorokiniana* of biomass reduce the $CO_2$ gas within a volume of 200 L, Tubular –photobioreactor 900 g/L, equivalent to 4.5 g dry weight of algae.

3. Reducing $CO_2$ through the use of the bioreactor. It was concluded that for every 1 g, of algae living mass, 1.7 g, of $CO_2$ is consumed.

4. The photobioreactor proved its efficiency in producing chemical compounds represented by proteins, Lipid and carbohydrates from *Chlorella sorokiniana* grown at a level of 25 L/min. of $CO_2$ gas, which reached 52, 35.6, and 14.3%, respectively, which is more than the laboratory experiment for the same level of adult gas 47.08% and 34.05% for proteins and lipids, respectively, despite the provision of all optimal environment conditions for development.

## Author details

Ahmed Aidan Al-Hussieny
Ministry of Higher Education and Scientific Research, Scientific Research Commission, Iraq

*Address all correspondence to: ahmed.edan85@gmail.com

## References

[1] Ekpo IJ. Slow response to climate change in Nigeria: Need for urgent and comprehensive action. Studies in Social Sciences and Humanities. 2014;**1**(1):19-29

[2] Pulz O, Broneske J, Waldeck P. IGV GmbH experience report, industrial production of microalgae under controlled conditions: Innovative prospects. In: Richmond A, Hu Q, editors. Handbook of Microalgal Culture: Applied Phycology and Biotechnology. 2nd ed. Oxford: Wiley; 2013. pp. 445-460

[3] Elliott LG, Feehan C, Laurens LML, Pienkos PT, Darzins A, Posewitz MC. Establishment of a bioenergy-focused microalgal culture collection. Algal Research. 2012;**1**:102-113

[4] Field CB, Behrenfeld MJ, Randerson JT, Falkowski P. Primary production of the biosphere: Integrating terrestrial and oceanic components. Science. 1998;**281**:237-240

[5] Chisti Y. Biodiesel from microalgae. Biotechnology Advances. 2007;**26**(3):294-306

[6] Lam MK, Lee KT. Effect of carbon source towards the growth of *Chlorella vulgaris* for $CO_2$ bio-mitigation and biodiesel production. International Journal of Greenhouse Gas Control. 2013;**14**:169-176

[7] Severo A, Deprá MC, Barin JS, Wagner R, de Menezes CR, Zepka LQ, et al. Bio-combustion of petroleum coke: The process integration with photobioreactors. Chemical Engineering Science. 2018;**177**:422-430

[8] Deprá C, Dias RR, Severo IA, de Menezes CR, Zepka LQ, Jacob-Lopes E. Carbon dioxide capture and use in photo bioreactors: The role of the carbon dioxide loads in the carbon footprint. Bioresource Technology. 2020;**314**:123745

[9] Rutherford JS, Wiegman AR, Day JW, Lane RR. Energy and climate–global trends and their implications for delta restoration. In: Mississippi Delta Restoration. Springer; 2018. pp. 77-92

[10] Owen NA, Inderwildi OR, King DA. The status of conventional world oil reserves—Hype or cause for concern? Energy Policy. 2010;**38**:4743-4749

[11] Singh S, Singh P. Effect of $CO_2$ concentration on algal growth: A review. Renewable and Sustainable Energy Reviews. 2014;**38**:172-179

[12] Stocker TF, Qin D, Plattner G-K, Tignor M, Allen SK, Boschung J, et al. IPCC, 2013: Climate Change 2013: The Physical Science Basis. Contribution of Working Group I to the Fifth Assessment Report of the Intergovernmental Panel on Climate Change. Cambridge University Press; 2013

[13] Kaithwas A, Prasad M, Kulshreshtha A, Verma S. Industrial wastes derived solid adsorbents for $CO_2$ capture: A mini review. Chemical Engineering Research and Design. 2012;**90**:1632-1641

[14] Krishnan B, Mudeva A. Palm Oil seen playing a role in EU Biofuels. Planet Ark. 2005. Available from: www.planetark.org/avantgo/daily newsstory.cfm.33265

[15] Alaswad A, Dassisti M, Prescott T, Olabi A. Technologies and developments of third generation biofuel production. Renewable and Sustainable Energy Reviews. 2015;**51**:1446-1460

[16] Hodaifa G, Martínez M, Sánchez S. Use of industrial wastewater from olive-oil extraction for biomass production of scenedesmus obliquus. Bioresource Technology. 2008;**99**(5):1111-1117

[17] Mata TM, Martins AA, Caetano NS. Microalgae for biodiesel production and other applications: A review. Renewable and Sustainable Energy Reviews. 2010;**14**(1):217-232

[18] Severo A, Siqueira SF, Deprá MC, Maroneze MM, Zepka LQ, Jacob-Lopes E. Biodiesel facilities: What can we address to make biorefineries commercially competitive. Renewable and Sustainable Energy Reviews. 2019;**112**:686-705

[19] Lardon L, Heỉlias A, Sialve B, Steyer JP, Bernard O. Life-cycle assessment of biodiesel production from microalgae. Environmental Science & Technology. 2009;**43**(17):6475-6481

[20] Tsukahara K, Sawayama S. Liquid fuel production using microalgae. Journal of the Japan Petroleum Institute. 2005;**48**(5):251-259

[21] Rodolfi L, Chini Zittelli G, Bassi N, Padovani G, Biondi N, Bonini G, et al. Microalgae for oil: Strain selection, induction of lipid synthesis and outdoor mass cultivation in a low-cost photo bioreactor. Biotechnology and Bioengineering. 2009;**102**(1):100-112

[22] Sambusiti C, Bellucci M, Zabaniotou A, Beneduce L, Monlau F. Algae as promising feedstocks for fermentative biohydrogen production according to a biorefinery approach: A comprehensive review. Renewable and Sustainable Energy Reviews. 2015;**44**:20-36

[23] Bharathiraja B, Chakravarthy M, Kumar RR, Yogendran D, Yuvaraj D, Jayamuthunagai J, et al. Aquatic biomass (algae) as a future feed stock for bio-refineries: A review on cultivation, processing and products. Renewable and Sustainable Energy Reviews. 2015;**47**:634-653

[24] Ziolkowska JR, Simon L. Recent developments and prospects for algae-based fuels in the US. Renewable and Sustainable Energy Reviews. 2014;**29**:847-853

[25] Chen C-Y, Kao P-C, Tan CH. Using an innovative pH-stat carbon dioxide feeding strategy to enhance cell growth and C-phycocyanin production from *Spirulina platensis*. Biochemical Engineering Journal. 2016;**112**:78-85

[26] Liu J, Huang J, Jiang Y, Chen F. Molasses-based growth and production of oil and astaxanthin by chlorella zofingiensis. Bioresource Technology. 2012;**107**:393-398

[27] Chen W-H, Lin B-J, Huang M-Y, Chang J-S. Thermochemical conversion of microalgal biomass into biofuels: A review. Bioresource Technology. 2015;**184**:314-327

[28] Al-Hussieny, Ahmed Aidan. Algae in Iraq its Environment and Classification, Place of Publication Ministry of Culture—Iraq. (Book in Arabic). 2017

[29] Abed IJ, Abdulhasan GA, Najem AM. Genotype versus phenotype to determine the definitive identification of the genera *chlorella* beijerinck, 1890 (chlorellaceae) and *Coelastrella.* Chodat, 1922 (scendesmaceae). Bulletin of the Iraq Natural History Museum. 2018;**15**:101-111. (P-ISSN: 1017-8678, E-ISSN: 2311-9799)

[30] Sims R, Taylor M. From 1st to 2st generation biofuel technologies. International Energy Agency (IEA Bioenergy). 2008:16-38

[31] Burton B. An OXFAM Hunger Banquet, Media Voices for Children, 04, 20. 2011. Available from: http://mediavoicesforchildren.org/?p=8573 [Accessed: April 20, 2013]

[32] Richmond A. Algae nutrition. In: Richmond A, editor. Handbook of Microalgae Culture: Biotechnology and Applied Phycology. Blackwell; 2004

[33] Cheah WY, Show PL, Chang JS, Ling TCJ, J.C. Biosequestration of atmospheric $CO_2$ and flue gas-containing $CO_2$ by microalgae. Bioresource Technology. 2015;**184**:190-201

[34] Moreira D, Pires. Atmospheric $CO_2$ capture by algae: Negative carbon dioxide emission path. Bioresource Technology. 2016;**215**:371-379

[35] Arbib Z, Ruiz J, Álvarez-Díaz P, Garrido-Pérez C, Perales JA. Capability of different microalgae species for phytoremediation processes: Wastewater tertiary treatment, $CO_2$ bio-fixation and low cost biofuels production. Water Research. 2014;**49**:465-474

[36] Li-Y CY, Chen P, Min M, Zhou W, Martinez B, Zhu J, et al. Characterization of a microalga *chlorella* sp. well adapted to highly concentrated municipal wastewater for nutrient removal and biodiesel production. Bioresource Technology. 2011;**102**:5138-5144

[37] Pandey JP, Tiwari A. Optimization of biomass production of Spirulina maxima. Journal of Algal Biomass Utilization. 2010;**1**(2):20-23

[38] Brown MR, Dunstan GA, Norwood SJ, Miller KA. Effects of harvest stage and light on the biochemical composition of the diatom *Thalassiosira pseudonana*. Journal of Phycology. 1996;**32**:64-73

[39] Kolb N, Vallaroni L, Milanovic N, Stocchi V. Evaluation of marine algae wakame (*Undaria pinnatifida*) and Kombu (*Laminaria digitata japonica*) as food suppliments. Food Technology and Biotechnology. 2004;**421**:57-67

[40] Spolaore P, Joannis-Cassan C, Duran E, Isambert A. Optimization of *Nannochloropsis oculata* growth using the response surface method. Journal of Chemical Technology and Biotechnology. 2006;**81**:1049-1056

[41] Gustafson KR, Oku N, Milanowski DJ. Anti-infective agents. Current Medicinal Chemistry. 2004;**3**:233

[42] Rasmussen RS, Morrissey MT. Marine biotechnology for production of food ingredients. Advances in Food and Nutrition Research. 2007;**52**:237-292

[43] Chen P, Min M, Chen Y, Wang L, Li Y, Chen Q, et al. Review of biological and engineering aspects of algae to fuels approach. International Journal of Agriculture and Biological Engineering. 2009;**2**(4):1-30

[44] Pereira S, Zille A, Micheletti E, Maradas-Ferreira P, De Phillipis R, Tumagnin P. Complexity of cyanobacterial expolyssacharides, composition structures, inducing factors and putative genes involved in their biosynthesis and assembly. FEM Microbiology Reviews. 2009;**33**(5):917-941

[45] Maroneze MM, Dias RR, Severo IA, Queiroz MI. Microalgae-Based Processes for Pigments Production. 2020. pp. 241-264

[46] Tredici MR, Chini Zittelli G, Rodolfi L. Photobioreactors. In: Flickinger MC, Anderson S, editors. Encyclopedia of Industrial Biotechnology: Bioprocess,

Bioseparation, and Cell Technology. Vol. 6. Hoboken: Wiley; 2010. pp. 3821-3838

[47] Acien Fernandez FG, Fernandez Sevilla JM, Molina Grima E. Photobioreactors for the production of microalgae. Reviews in Environmental Science and Biotechnology. 2013;**12**:131-151

[48] Masojídek J, Papáček S, Sergejevová M, Jirka V, Červený C, Kunc J, et al. A closed solar photobioreactor for cultivation of microalgae under supra-high irradiance: Basic design and performance. Journal of Applied Phycology. 2003;**15**:239-248

[49] Masojídek J, Sergejevová M, Rottnerová K, Jirka V, Korečko J, Kopecký J, et al. A two-stage solar photobioreactor for cultivation of microalgae based on solar concentrators. Journal of Applied Phycology. 2009;**21**:55-63

[50] Singh UB, Ahluwalia AS. Microalgae: A promising tool for carbon sequestration. Mitigation and Adaptation Strategies for Global Change. 2013;**18**(1). DOI: 10.1007/s11027-012-9393-3

[51] Vo TS, Kim SK. Potential anti-HIV agents from marine resources: An overview. Marine Drugs. 2010;**8**:2871-2892

[52] Baumler ER, Crapiste GH, Carelli AA. Solvent extraction: Kinetic study of major and minor compounds. Journal of the American Oil Chemists' Society. 2010;**87**:1489-1495

[53] Giannelli L, Torzillo G. Hydrogen production with the microalga *Chlamydomonas reinhardtii* grown in a compact tubular photobioreactor immersed in a scattering nanoparticle suspension. International Journal of Hydrogen Energy. 2012;**37**:16951-16961

[54] Becker, Howard S. Telling About Society. Chicago: University of Chicago Press; 2007

Chapter 4

# An Overview of the Importance of Macroalgae in the Aquaculture Industry

*Vahid Morshedi*

## Abstract

The increase in the price of fish meal, as well as the decrease in its availability, has led to a rapidly expanding search for suitable herbal alternatives over the years. Macroalgae are a good alternative because of their easy growth and reasonable price. Macroalgae are used as dietary supplements to enhance the health, growth, and feeding performance of many species of marine and freshwater fish, as well as ornamental fish. Most studies have reported acceptable results in using macroalgae as a relative alternative to fish meal. Meanwhile, the amount of crude protein and polysaccharides in red macrophages is higher than in other species. The results show that although the use of algae flour by up to 10% in the culture of some species, such as red seabream (*Pagrus major*), European sea bass (*Dicentrarchus labraxa*), and Asian sea bass (Lates calcarifer) has increased growth and feeding performance, using more from algae flour in the diet of some species, the difference was not observed between treatments and even had negative effects. Therefore, it seems that more research is needed in this field.

**Keywords:** aquaculture, macroalgae, fish diet, Persian gulf, marine fish

## 1. Introduction

Aquatic animals are considered one of the main sources of human food [1]. Currently, the global per capita consumption of seafood is estimated at 20 kilograms, with nearly half of it supplied by farmed seafood [2]. On the other hand, considering the advancements in the aquaculture industry in recent decades, a significant portion of the global catch has been allocated for the production of fish meal and oil as raw materials in the formulation of aquaculture feed. Considering the global increase in demand for fish meal and oil production and the estimated aquaculture production growth rate of 6.5% annually until 2025, it is predicted that, in a short period, aquaculture will consume all the produced fish meal and oil [3]. Moreover, it is predicted that, in the future, due to the depletion of ocean reserves and the increase in the price of fish meal and oil, the development of the aquaculture industry will be significantly limited, and consequently, maintaining the status and sustainability of the aquaculture industry will be difficult solely by using these resources [4]. Therefore, any substitution of this expensive material (fish meal), even in low percentages, can have a significant impact on reducing the cost of feed and the produced product. Unfortunately, for various reasons, in many cases, the catch of low-quality aquatic animals has been on the agenda of fish meal production factories [5]. Therefore, the use of alternative sources in fish feed should be considered and discussed.

The aquaculture industry, particularly seaweed cultivation, is rapidly growing. Currently, these algae are cultivated in 50 countries worldwide, and among the groups of farmed aquatic animals, seaweeds hold the largest share, with a volume of approximately 27 million tons [2]. Among the nutrients, the levels of protein and fat are important factors that make them an ideal supplement for the diets of aquatic animals. Protein is one of the most expensive and important components of the aquatic diet. The protein content of macroalgae has been reported to be in the range of 5–40 percent of dry weight (in a few cases, more than 40 percent). At the same time, their fat content has been recorded at only 2–5 percent of dry weight. Despite the low total fat content, a significant portion of these fat sources includes unsaturated fatty acids, which seem essential for the growth and development of aquatic organisms, especially during the larval and juvenile stages. In addition to the aforementioned factors, the presence of vitamins, minerals, pigments, antioxidants, and some polysaccharides with the ability to bind minerals plays an important role in nutritional balance and growth improvement in diets containing macroalgae [6]. Most of the conducted studies have reported satisfactory results in using macroalgae as a partial substitute for fish meal. Various studies have shown that the impact of using macroalgae in the diets of aquatic animals depends on the type of algae used, the species of fish studied, and the level of substitution [7].

## 2. The importance of macroalgae

Cultivating seaweed can serve as an economical and profitable activity, especially for coastal communities, as its production cycle is short, it requires low investment, and its cultivation technology is relatively simple. On the one hand, macroalgae grow abundantly in their natural habitat, which is the seas and oceans. On the other hand, the shallow coastal waters around the world are rich in nutrients and pollutants, which are caused by ecosystem activities such as coastal currents and upwelling or by agricultural activities and wastewater discharge along the shores. Cultivating algae in these areas can act as an environmentally friendly activity that absorbs these nutrients. In addition to the aforementioned points, seaweed cultivation, unlike agricultural activities conducted on land that require large volumes of freshwater, can reduce pressure on water resources and agricultural production without the need for freshwater [6]. Approximately 300 species of seaweeds have been identified in the southern part of the country, classified into the categories of red algae (Rhodophytes), brown algae (Phaeophytes), and green algae (Chlorophytes) [8]. The most important cultivated seaweeds in the world are *Echeuma spp.*, *Saccharina spp.*, *Gracilaria spp.*, *Undaria spp.*, and Porphyra spp. Among the notable and important characteristics of algae that have made their use as supplements or one of the main items in the diet of aquatic animals significant are their richness in bioactive substances, proteins, and carbohydrates, which are essential components of the diet for humans and animals. On the other hand, algae contain a high percentage of fatty acids, making their use in the diets of aquatic animals very important and vital [9].

Macro and microalgae are used as dietary supplements to enhance the health and nutritional performance of many cultured fish species [10]. Macroalgae, compared to microalgae, contain less protein; however, their use has significantly impacted growth improvement, fat metabolism, and meat quality enhancement [11]. Macroalgae also contain proteins, carbohydrates (starch, glucose, sugars, and indigestible polysaccharides such as agar, carrageenan, and alginate), fats (glycerol and fatty acids of the n-3 (omega-3) and n-6 (omega-6) series with antibacterial, antiviral, and antifungal properties), essential vitamins (A, B1, B2, B6, B12, C, E, biotin, folic acid, and pantothenic acid), minerals (phosphorus, zinc, iron, calcium, selenium, and manganese), and antioxidants [12]. The color of the skin or flesh of fish is an important characteristic in the aquaculture industry, which creates an attractive appearance and consequently satisfies consumers. In this regard, the presence of natural pigments in macroalgae and their use in fish feed can create an effective color in the flesh and skin [6]. Improvement in growth, feed consumption, liver function, fat metabolism, physiological activities, stress responses, disease resistance, and meat quality has been reported in diets containing 1–5% macroalgae. Additionally, some reports have recommended adding a mixture of macroalgae to the diet instead of using a single species of macroalgae, which results in improved growth performance and better fish taste [9].

Despite the aforementioned points confirming the high nutritional value of macroalgae and their positive effects on the health of aquatic animals and humans, it should be noted that algae also have specific challenges, and caution should be exercised before using them in the diets of aquatic animals or humans. For example, among more than 200,000 species of algae, only less than 20 percent have been reported as nontoxic. Many species of algae contain heavy metals (mercury, lead, and arsenic), and in some cases, their concentration exceeds that of the surrounding environment. Additionally, some species of algae capable of producing toxins have been reported, which may cause neurological disorders in the host organism by producing biogenic toxins and secondary metabolites [6].

## 3. Biochemical compounds of macroalgae

The biochemical composition of macroalgae varies significantly between species, harvest season, growth habitat, and environmental conditions. Even in a small geographical area, the growth rate and biochemical compositions of macroalgae may vary depending on the harvest season, sunlight, salinity, depth, and local water flow. Reports have shown that the biochemical composition of algae can even have significant differences within similar genera of algae. The biochemical composition of some macroalgae is presented in **Table 1** [13].

Macroalgae contain high amounts of essential minerals (10–50 percent of dry weight), including calcium, magnesium, potassium, and sodium, as well as trace elements (copper, manganese, zinc, and iron) that play an important role in the formation of tissues in organisms and as cofactors in regulating many vital reactions. Algae, due to their possession of surface polysaccharides (such as agar, carrageenan, alginate, and cellulose) are capable of absorbing minerals from the environment. Accordingly, the mineral content in macroalgae may be several times higher than the similar elements present in the ecosystem. The number of mineral elements in macroalgae can also vary depending on the type of algae, seasonal changes, geographical location, and light intensity [6]. Macroalgae contain relatively low amounts of fat, but

| Chemical constituent [a] | Brown macroalgae [b] | Green macroalgae [c] | Red macroalgae [d] |
|---|---|---|---|
| Wet biomass | 610–940 | 780–920 | 720–910 |
| Crude protein [e] | 24–168 | 33–352 | 64–376 |
| Crude lipids | 3–96 | 3–28 | 2–129 |
| Polysaccharides | 380–610 | 150–650 | 360–660 |
| Ash | 150–450 | 110–550 | 120–422 |

[a] *Values are in g/kg of dry matter (DM) unless otherwise specified.*
[b] *Values are for typical brown macroalgal species: e.g., Laminaria, Sac-charina, Fucus, Ascophyllum, Alaria, Pelvetia, and Undaria spp.*
[c] *Values are for typical green macroalgal species: e.g., Ulva, Cladophora, and Enteromorpha spp.*
[d] *Values are for typical red macroalgal species: e.g., Palmaria, Chondrus, Porphyra, Vertebrata, and Gracilaria spp.*
[e] *All values for crude protein (CP) have been recalculated using the recommended nitrogen-to-protein factor of five.*

**Table 1.**
*Ranges of proximate composition of marine macroalgae.*

fats are highly important due to their unsaturated fatty acids. Eicosapentaenoic acid (EPA) and docosahexaenoic acid (DHA) are considered among the most important polyunsaturated fatty acids (HUFA) due to their numerous applications in the diets of all life stages of aquatic animals, including larvae, juvenile fish, grow-out fish, and broodstock, as well as their medicinal applications. Research shows that the presence of polyunsaturated fatty acids in fish oil is derived from the consumption of phyto-plankton by zooplankton and through the marine food chain. Therefore, research on the direct use of macroalgae in the diets of aquatic animals to enhance the levels of polyunsaturated fatty acids in fish has begun. Lee et al. [14] reported an increase in the level of polyunsaturated fatty acids along with weight gain and feed consump-tion in catfish, even with very low amounts (1–1.5 percent). However, the results of studies indicate that due to the low level of EPA in seaweeds, they cannot be used as a substitute for polyunsaturated fatty acids in fish diets [6].

## 4. Protein and amino acid content of macroalgae

The protein content in macroalgae ranges from 5 to 40 percent of dry weight and varies across different seasons and species. Generally, the highest protein content is obtained during winter and early spring, while the lowest amount is found in summer and early autumn. In general, red algae have a low protein content compared to brown macroalgae (usually less than 150 grams per kilogram of dry matter), while green macroalgae, and especially red macroalgae, have a higher protein content [15]. Some red macroalgae, such as Porphyra (*Porphyra* sp.), have a protein content comparable to that of soy powder [16]. The comparison of different protein results of macroal-gae in conducted studies may be due to various measurement methods. Nitrogen is found in proteins, nucleic acids, and several organic compounds, such as chlorophyll. Additionally, macroalgae themselves contain significant amounts of non-protein-aceous mineral nitrogen (e.g., ammonia, nitrate, and nitrite). Spectroscopic methods are often used to determine protein content, but many proteins in macroalgae can be extracted and contain several colored substances that may affect the measurement [17]. However, for nutritional purposes, amino acid analysis of the algae must be conducted. Another challenging issue regarding the protein content of macroalgae relates to the complete digestion of algal protein by aquatic organisms or other

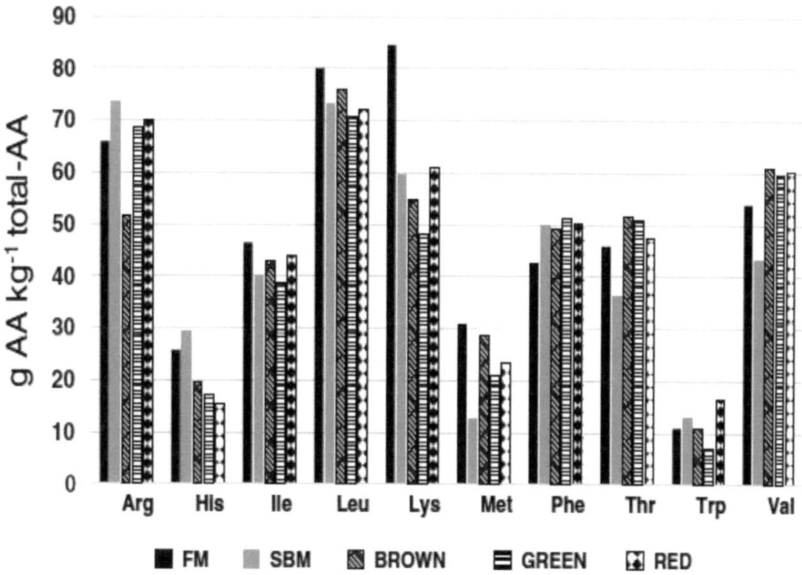


**Figure 1.**
*Typical essential amino acid (EAA) profiles of fishmeal (FM), soybean meal (SBM) and brown, green, and red marine macroalgae. Values are averages for the most common macroalgal species reported in the literature expressed as g AA $kg^{-1}$ of total AA for each EAA [18].*

creatures. Despite the high protein content in macroalgae, not all protein components of the algae are biologically significant. About 10 percent of the crude protein consists of nonprotein substances such as amines, nucleic acids, and nitrogen-containing cell walls. The protein in macroalgae contains all amino acids, including glycine, arginine, alanine, and glutamic acid. The levels of essential amino acids in macroalgae are comparable to the protein requirements stated by FAO and WHO [13]. A general comparison of the ratio of essential amino acids in fish meal, soybean meal, red algae, green algae, and brown algae is presented in **Figure 1** [13].

## 5. The carbohydrate content of macroalgae

Carbohydrates are biomolecules composed of carbon, hydrogen, and oxygen atoms, and they are classified into three forms: monosaccharides, oligosaccharides, and polysaccharides. Macroalgae are now used as a rich source of carbohydrates in various industries. Among red algae, *Gracilaria sp.* and *Hypnea* sp. have been studied more due to its polysaccharides, such as agar and carrageenan (with multiple medicinal uses). On the other hand, green and brown algae contain significant amounts of polysaccharides and other carbohydrates, as shown in **Table 2**. Macroalgae, due to their high content of indigestible polysaccharides, are usually recognized as suitable sources of fiber (30–60 percent of dry weight). Among the fibers, hydrocolloids such as alginate, agar, carrageenan, fucoidan, and laminarin are present in large quantities in algae. Fiber is usually attributed to the indigestible carbohydrates in food. These compounds pass through the digestive system intact and will be fermented at the end of the intestine. Some of the polysaccharides that pass through the cell wall and are soluble in water are referred to as soluble fiber, while those that pass through the entire digestive tract and reach the end of the intestine are referred to as insoluble

| **Chemical constituent** [a] | **Brown macroalgae** | **Green macroalgae** | **Red macroalgae** |
|---|---|---|---|
| Polysaccharides | alginate, laminarin, fucoidan (sulphated), cellulose, mannitol | ulvan (sulphated), mannan, galactans (sulphated), xylans, starch, cellulose, lignin | Carrageenans (sulphated), agar (sulphated), glucans (floridean starch), cellulose, lignin, funoran |
| Monosaccharides | Glucose, galactose,fucose, xylose, uronic acid, mannuronic acid, guluronic acid, glucuronic acid | Glucose, mannose, rhamnose, xylose, uronic acid, glucuronic acid | Glucose, galactose, agarose |
| Total fiber | 170–690 | 290–670 | 150–590 |
| Soluble fiber | 257–370 | 170–240 | 80-370 |
| Insoluble fiber | 47–400 | 160–190 | 80–270 |

*Values in grams per kilogram.*
[a] *Values in specific red, brown, and green algae.*

**Table 2.**
*Description and content range of carbohydrates in marine macroalgae [18]*.*

fiber. The former increases viscosity in the intestine, and the latter increases stool volume and reduces transit time. Therefore, when macroalgae are used in the diet, fiber is an important component of it. In the **Table 2** below, Orland et al. [13] have shown that, on average, soluble fiber, insoluble fiber, and total fiber in red algae species are lower than in green and brown types [13]. The number of polysaccharides in algae is influenced by several factors, including biological, physical, and environmental factors. For example, the harvesting time, species of algae, and the guidelines and methods of polysaccharide extraction may affect its quantity and structure. This issue significantly affects the performance and properties of polysaccharides [19].

## 6. The application of macroalgae in fish diets

Since the 1960s, extensive research has been conducted to obtain inexpensive protein sources for feeding the growing human population as well as animals, including aquatic species. Since fish meal is the most abundant yet the most expensive source of animal protein in the production of poultry, livestock, and aquaculture feed, global markets have always been in search of a suitable alternative [20]. Alternative plant and animal sources for fish meal, such as soybean meal, flaxseed meal, corn gluten meal, squid meal, shrimp meal, bone and meat meal, hydrolyzed feather meal, blood meal, and poultry by-products, have been investigated in various studies for partial or complete replacement of fish meal; however, even these protein sources will not be sufficient for the growing aquaculture industry [21]. Despite extensive research conducted, a suitable animal or plant protein source that can completely replace fish meal has not yet been reported. As mentioned, reducing dependence on fish meal is possible, but completely replacing fish meal with other substitutes without affecting the growth performance of fish and shrimp is impossible [22] regarding the replacement of fish meal with plant proteins such as soy, rapeseed, corn, etc. In the diets of farmed aquatic animals, extensive research has been conducted worldwide, and valuable results and various optimal levels have been reported. In this context, most research has focused on replacing fish meal with soybean meal, and less research has been conducted on other plant proteins, including seaweeds. On the other hand, the deficiencies in the amino acid profile and the presence of certain anti-nutritional factors in most agricultural products limit their use, and today, researchers are using technology to eliminate these anti-nutritional factors [5].

The use of seaweed meal in animal and aquaculture feed was first introduced in Norway in 1960, where dried and ground brown seaweeds were used in aquaculture feed. Additionally, Mostafa and colleagues, after the Norwegians, highlighted the importance of macroalgae as food items in fish diets in 1995. Subsequently, several studies were conducted to utilize marine macroalgae (Sargassum, Porphyra, Ulva, Gracilaria, and Padina) in the diets of aquatic animals, some of which will be mentioned below.

In a study, Morshedi et al. [23] reported that the inclusion of *Gracilaria pulvinata* in the diet of Asian sea bass (*Lates calcarifer*) affected blood and immune parameters but did not impact the fish's body composition. In this study, a diet containing 3% *Gracilaria pulvinata* showed better effects on growth performance, body composition, and health parameters of the fish [23]. In another study on Asian sea bass, replacing macroalgae *Kappaphycus alvarezii*, *Eucheuma denticulatum*, and *Sargassum polycystum* at a level of 5% did not show significant differences in growth parameters [24]. The study by Solar Villa et al. [25] also showed that the amount of the red macroalga Porphyra dioica had a negative effect on the growth of rainbow trout (*Oncorhynchus mykiss*) at a level of 15%. However, at a level of 10%, the replacement of Porphyra macroalga did not negatively affect growth and nutrition performance and improved the fish's body composition and flesh color in terms of pigment content. Also, Pham et al. [26] reported that the use of 6% Hizikia fusiformis macroalgae powder in the diet of olive flounder (*Paralichthys olivaceus*) increased growth performance compared to the other treatments (0%, 2%, and 4% levels). The results of the study by Wassef [27] on two macroalgae, *Ulva lactuca* and *Pterocladia capillacea*, showed that the use of 5% of these two macroalgae in the diet of sea bass (*Dicentrarchus labrax*) improved growth and increased survival. Additionally, the results of the study by Mostafa et al. [28] on the red sea bream (*Pagrus major*) showed that feeding with three types of macroalgae such as *Ascophyllum nodosum*, *Porphyra yezoensis*, and *Ulva pertusa* at a rate of 5% improved growth. In most conducted studies, replacing macroalgae by 5–10% has had a positive and significant impact, while at higher levels, the growth and nutritional performance of fish were negatively and significantly affected [7]. This trend has been reported in various studies [29], and the reason is the reduced digestibility of protein and fat due to the anti-nutritional properties of soluble non-starch polysaccharides in algae, which increase with the percentage of macroalgae in the diet. Non-starch polysaccharides reduce the digestion and absorption of nutrients by inhibiting the activity of digestive enzymes or binding to bile acids.

## 7. Conclusion

Since nutrition plays an important role in the growth of aquatic animals, using an appropriate diet can significantly contribute to meeting their nutritional needs. In general, macroalgae have a high potential for use as a supplement or raw material in the diets of aquatic animals and other animals. However, their commercial use depends more on initial access to the raw product and the quality of the product in terms of biochemical composition. In addition, the use of the potential of macroalgae in the aquaculture diet and the costs involved in their production, harvesting, and processing before use in fish feed depend on comparisons with currently used products in the diets. In this regard, limiting factors that reduce and even prevent the digestion and consumption of macroalgae by aquatic animals should be identified in various studies, and their nutritional and physiological effects in the long term should be evaluated. Most of the conducted studies have reported satisfactory results in using macroalgae as a partial substitute for fish meal (up to a maximum of 10 percent). However, research results have shown that the impact of using macroalgae in the diets of aquatic animals depends on the type of algae used, the species of fish studied, and the level of substitution. Therefore, for each species of cultured fish, the type and amount of algae should be studied.

## Acknowledgements

This chapter is an English translation of a previously published work in the Iranian Journal of Biology (DOI: https://dor.isc.ac/dor/20.1001.1.20089406.1400.5.10.13.1). Link: https://www.ijbio.ir/article_2017.

## Author details

Vahid Morshedi
Persian Gulf Research Institution, Persian Gulf University, Iran

*Address all correspondence to: v.morshedi@gmail.com; v.morshedi@pgu.ac.ir

## References

[1] Ayoola AA. Replacement of fish meal with alternative protein source in aquaculture diets [thesis]. North Carolina, USA: North California State University; 2010

[2] FAO. The State of World Fisheries and Aquaculture 2016-Meeting the Sustainable Development Goals. Rome, Italy: FAO; 2016

[3] Collins SA, Shand PJ, Drew MD. Stabilization of linseed oil with vitamin E, butylated hydroxytoluene, and lipid encapsulation affects fillet lipid composition and sensory characteristics when fed to rainbow trout. Animal Feed Science and Technology. 2011;**170**:53-62

[4] Bouraoui L, Sánchez-Gurmaches J, Cruz-Garcia L, Gutiérrez J, Benedito-Palos L, Pérez-Sánchez J, et al. Effect of dietary fish meal and fish oil replacement on lipogenic and lipoprotein lipase activities and plasma insulin in gilthead sea bream (*Sparus auratus*). Aquaculture Nutrition. 2011;**17**:54-63

[5] Hardy RW. Aquaculture's rapid growth requirements for alternative protein sources. Feed Management Journal. 1999;**50**:25-28

[6] Tiwari BK, Troy DJ. Seaweed Sustainability. New York, USA: Academic Press, Elsevier Science; 2015. p. 472

[7] Pereira R, Valente LMP, Sousa-Pinto I, Rema P. Apparent nutrient digestibility of seaweeds by rainbow trout (*Oncorhynchus mykiss*) and Nile tilapia (*Oreochromis niloticus*). Algal Research. 2012;**1**:77-82

[8] Gharanjik B, Abkenar A. Identification of seaweed in Sistan and Baluchestan Province costal zone. Iranian Scientific Fisheries Journal. 1999;**9**:37-48

[9] Nakagawa H, Montgomery WL. Algae. In: Nakagawa H, Sato M, Gatlin DM III, editors. Dietary Supplements for the Health and Quality of Cultured Fish. Cambridge, USA: CABI International; 2007. pp. 133-167

[10] Güroy D, Güroy B, Merrifield DL, Ergün S, Tekinay AA, Yiğit M. Effect of dietary Ulva and spirulina on weight loss and body composition of rainbow trout, *Oncorhynchus mykiss* (Walbaum), during a starvation period. Journal of Animal Physiology and Animal Nutrition. 2011;**95**:320-327

[11] Wassef EA, Elmasry MH, Mikhail FR. Growth enhancement and muscle structure of striped mullet, *Mugil cephalus* L., fingerlings by feeding algal meal-based diets. Aquaculture Research. 2001;**32**:315-322

[12] Kumar CS, Ganesan P, Suresh PV, Bhaskar N. Seaweeds as a source of nutritionally beneficial compounds- a review. Journal Food Science Technology. 2008;**45**:1-13

[13] Øverland M, Mydland LT, Skrede A. Marine macroalgae as a source of protein and bioactive compounds in feed for monogastric animals. Norwegian University of Life Sciences. 2019;**99**(1):13-24

[14] Li MH, Robinson EH, Tucker CS, Manning BB, Khoo L. Effects of dried algae *Schizochytrium* sp., a rich source of docosahexaenoic acid, on growth, fatty acid composition, and sensory quality of channel catfish *Ictalurus punctatus*. Aquaculture. 2009;**292**:232-236

[15] Garcia-Vaquero M, Hayes M. Red and green macroalgae for fish and animal feed and human functional

food development. Food Reviews International. 2016;**32**(1):15-45

[16] Smith JL, Summers G, Wong R. Nutrient and heavy metal content of edible seaweeds in New Zealand. New Zealand Journal of Crop and Horticultural Science. 2010;**38**:19-28

[17] Angell AR, Mata L, de Nys R, Paul NA. The protein content of seaweeds: A universal nitrogen-to-protein conversion factor of five. Journal of Applied Phycology. 2016;**28**(1):511-524

[18] Øverland M, Mydland LT, Skrede A. Marine macroalgae as sources of protein and bioactive compounds in feed for monogastric animals. Journal of the Science of Food and Agriculture. 2019;**99**(1):13-24

[19] Holdt SL, Kraan S. Bioactive compounds in seaweed: Functional food applications and legislation. Journal of Applied Phycology. 2011;**23**:543-597

[20] Ferraz de Arruda L, Borghesi R, Oetterer M. Use of fish waste as silage - a review. Brazilian Archives of Biology and Technology. 2007;**50**:879-886

[21] Rangacharyulu PV, Giri SS, Paul BN, Yashoda KP, Rao RJ, Mahendrakar NS, et al. Utilization of fermented silkworm pupae silage in feed for carps. Bioresource Technology. 2003;**86**:29-32

[22] Makkar HPS, Tran G, Heuze V, Giger-Reverdin S, Lessire M, Lebas F, et al. Seaweeds for livestock diets: A review. Animal Feed Science and Technology. 2016;**212**:1-17

[23] Morshedi V, Nafisi Bahabadi M, Sotoudeh E, Azodi M, Hafezieh M. Nutritional evaluation of *Gracilaria pulvinata* as partial substitute with fish meal in practical diets of barramundi (*Lates calcarifer*). Journal of Applied Phycology. 2018;**30**(1):619-628

[24] Shapawi R, Zamry AA. Response of Asian seabass, *Lates calcarifer* juvenile fed with different seaweed-based diets. Journal of Applied Animal Research. 2016;**44**(1):121-125

[25] Soler-Vila A, Coughlan S, Guiry MD, Stefan K. The red algae *Porphyra dioicaas* a fish-feed ingredient for rainbow trout (*Oncorhynchus mykiss*): Effects on growth, feed efficiency, and carcass composition. Journal of Applied Phycology. 2009;**21**:617-624

[26] Pham MA, Lee KJ, Lee BJ, Lim SJ, Kim SS, Lee YD, et al. Effects of dietary *Hizikia fusiformis* on growth and immune responses in juvenile olive flounder (*Paralichthys olivaceus*). Asian-Australasian Journal of Animal Sciences. 2006;**19**(12):1769-1775

[27] Wassef EA. Alternative protein sources for fish feeds in Egypt. Cahiers Options Méditerranéennes. 2005;**63**:127-141

[28] Mustafa G, Wakamatsufa S, Takeda T, Umino T, Nakagawa H. Effects of algae meal as feed additive on growth, feed efficiency, and body composition in red sea bream. Fisheries Science. 1995;**61**(1):25-28

[29] Hasan MR, Chakrabarti R. Use of Algae and Aquatic Macrophytes as Feed in Small-Scale Aquaculture: A Review. Rome: Food and Agriculture Organization of the United Nations; 2009

Chapter 5

# Microalgae and Seaweeds as Feed Additives for Aquatic Animals: Effects on Growth, Immunity, and Disease Resistance

*Einar Ringø, Mohamed Ashour, Sherine Ahmed, Zaki Sharawy, Ashraf Goda and Ehab El-Haroun*

## Abstract

Algae and derivatives are currently being recognized for their potential characteristics as attributes in aquafeeds. These include their high protein content, optimum balance of essential amino acids and fatty acids, trace minerals, vitamins, and relatively low cost, which make them promising alternatives in the diets of farmed fish and shrimp. The inclusion of algae and their bioactive compounds in fish diets provides natural sources of growth promoters and immunostimulants, which improve growth and immune system response and mitigate disease outbreaks and pathogen infections. However, too much substitution would result in poor development and feed utilization. Therefore, this chapter discusses the forms and types of algae, their use in fish feed, the pros and cons of algae, which aid in achieving aquaculture sustainability and their scope for practical implementation.

**Keywords:** aquaculture, algae, feed supplements, fish, shellfish, shrimp

## 1. Introduction

Aquaculture currently represents half of the world's animal protein supply, but several challenges face the expansion of the global aquaculture industry and fisheries [1, 2]. These include issues such as pollution and climate change, high aquafeed production costs with low quality, unstable water supply, low immunity, and widespread fish diseases [3–5]. These challenges are pressuring scientists and researchers into doing more research looking for novel ingredients and feed additives to control these problems and limit their negative impacts on aquaculture industry that consequently impact the sustainability of aquaculture and fisheries [6]. Therefore, to guarantee the sustainability of aquaculture, these problems must be solved through maintainable and environmentally friendly applications [7, 8]. Feed quality and meeting nutritional requirements are major issues, affecting fish growth and overall health [9, 10]. Since aquafeeds account for 50 to 80 percent of aquaculture production costs, their use should be properly regulated [11]. Expansion of the aquafeed industry is expected to reach 8–10% annually, and by 2025, 73.15 million tonnes of feed will be produced to meet demand [12]. Aquaculture feeds consume approximately 55% of forage fish caught annually worldwide [13]. Nowadays, considerable research is being conducted to find alternative ingredients to replace fish meal and fish oil in aquafeeds due to the decline in fishmeal and oil production for aquafeeds [14–16]. As such, several strategies have been recently applied to sustain and develop aquaculture production [17]. Therefore, the utilization of feed additives has emerged as a primary strategy in aquaculture [18]. Many feed additives have been used in aqua diets such as algae derivatives, algae extract, binders, antimicrobials, antioxidants, enzymes, immunostimulants, prebiotics, and probiotics [13, 19–26]. Due to their high content of bioactive molecules [19], algae are frequently used in several bioindustries including food supplements [27, 28], wastewater treatment [29–33], biofertilizers [25], antimicrobial activities [34], and aquaculture feed additives [26]. The aquaculture industry now has a great opportunity to exploit various aquatic plants like weeds, and microalgae due to their high content of bioactive compounds and providing a cheap source of protein available for aquafeeds available [35]. Studies have shown that algae possess a highly digestible protein, balance, and available amino acids versus other sources of proteins, offering a chance to enhance and improve feed quality [36, 37]. In addition, the presence of bioactive compounds in algae and seaweed aids to enhance the immunity of fish and shrimp; thus, the inclusion of algae and seaweeds serves as an ideal ingredient that can improve health and welfare [6, 21].

Furthermore, the inclusion of macroalgae and seaweeds in fish and shrimp diets has a significant impact on reducing feed costs [24]. In summary, algae have been shown to enhance growth, immune response, and disease resistance when included in aquatic animal production diets. Therefore, this chapter discusses the types of algae, their use in fish feed, and their effects on growth and various physiological responses. Furthermore, it discusses the pros and cons of using algae in feed to achieve aquaculture sustainability.

## 2. Types of algae

There are two types of algae: seaweed (macroalgae) and microalgae, which are important sources of protein [38, 39]. They are similar in nutritional composition to soybeans and other plant proteins, making them a viable option for sustainable biomass production in aquaculture as well as many other applications for animal production [40, 41].

### 2.1 Macroalgae (seaweeds)

Macroalgae are recognized with various advantages in comparison to land plants, including the ability to be grown without the need for freshwater, fertilizer, pesticides, or arable land, and the biomass's potential for use as materials, food, feed, gelling agents, and bioenergy [39, 42]. In addition, microalgae and seaweeds are rich in bioactive compounds such as peptides, phenols, and polysaccharides, as well as a wide range of carbohydrates (such as oligosaccharides) and antioxidants like beta-carotene, vitamins (C, D, and E), and different polyphenols [43–46]. Therefore, microalgae and seaweed are becoming more and more popular for fish nutrition [36].

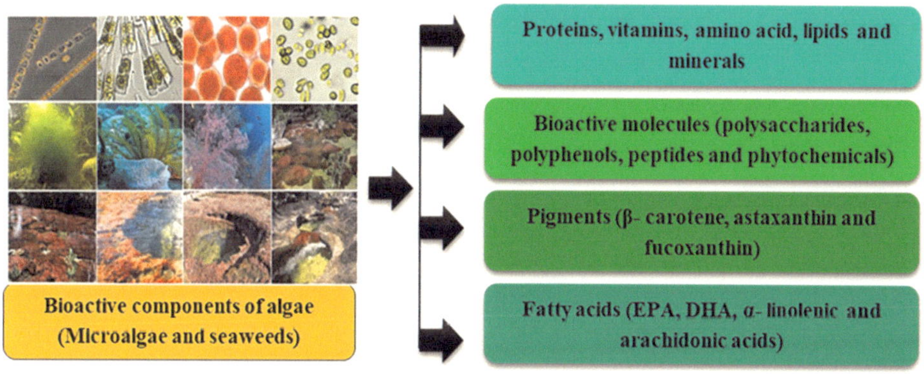


**Figure 1.**
*Bioactive components of algae (micro and macroalgae).*

In addition, it has functional characteristics such as prebiotic substances like β-glucan and oligosaccharides. They also have a lot of minerals, vitamins, and PUFAs that are good for health, growth, bone development, and immune response [47], and gut microbiota [48], which may enhance nutrient assimilation, thereby promoting fish growth performance [36]. Seaweeds are categorized into three groups based on color: green, brown algae, and red algae. Several studies showed that the use of algae, seaweed, and extracts enhances growth, growth, and immune-related gene expression and controls pathogen infections and disease outbreaks of various fish and crustaceans, such as gilthead sea bream, European sea bass *Dicentrarchus labrax* [49], Pacific white shrimp, *Litopenaeus vannamei* [19], banana shrimp, *Fenneropenaeus merguiensis* [50], Asian Seabass, *Lates calcarifer* [51], Nile Tilapia, *Oreochromis niloticus* [52], and Rainbow Trout, *Oncorhynchus mykiss* [53].

### *2.1.1 Seaweed chemical composition and bioactive compounds*

Many factors affect the nutrient chemical composition of seaweeds, including species, growing habitat, harvest age, season, location, temperature, salinity, and species (**Figure 1**, [29]), and they contain varying amounts of ash (7–38%), high amounts of CHO (up to 60%), low quantities of fat (1–3%), and high quantities of proteins (10–47%) [30], with an excellent combination of EAAs, vitamins, minerals and fiber [31].

Additionally, algae contain a variety of bioactive substances, such as phenols, and polysaccharides; pigmentation, vitamin C, and an array of CHOs as oligosaccharides [16]. These products support the growth of probiotics, resulting in higher growth performance, immune system, and pathogen infection in fish [32]. **Table 1** shows the chemical composition of different types of seaweed.

## 2.2 Microalgae

Microalgae are also recognized for their high content of bioactive compounds [64]. Microalgae have dual functions: (i) low-cost water treatment and (ii) provide high-value biomass as a nutritious and sustainable feed source in aquaculture nutrition [65]. In addition, they act as growth promoters, anti-inflammatory, antibacterial, and immunostimulants, enhancing the growth and immune response of farmed fish [7].

| Macroalgae spices | Biochemical composition (%, dry weight bases) | | | References |
|---|---|---|---|---|
| | Proteins | Lipids | Carbohydrates | |
| **Red seaweeds (Rhodophyceae)** | | | | |
| *Ahnfeltia plicata* | 20.1–31.1 | 1.1 | 30.2–59.1 | [54, 55] |
| *Gracilaria cervicornis* | 19.70 | 0.43 | 64 | [56] |
| *Pterocladia capillacea* | 17–20 | 47–51 | 1.7–2.5 | [57] |
| *Porphyra tenera* | 36.6–47 | 3.1 | 36.6–37 | [58] |
| *Kappaphycus Alvarezii* | 16.24 | 0.74 | 27.40 | [59] |
| **Brown seaweeds (Phaeophyta)** | | | | |
| *Spatoglossum schroederi* | 5–21 | 1.6–2.3 | 0.1–59.3 | [60] |
| *Ascophyllum nodosum* | 5.9–8.5 | 2–2.65 | 31.7–59 | [61] |
| *Spatoglossum schroederi* | 5.21–21.5 | 3.1 | 40.1–59.3 | [60] |
| *Laurencia obtusa* | 21 | 3 | 4 | [57] |
| *Undaria pinnatifida* | 12.5–15.7 | 2.2 | 55.9 | [62] |
| *Cystoseira compressa* | 9.98 | 2.80 | 39.11 | [55] |
| *Colpomenia sinuosa* | 9.20 | 1.50 | 32.10 | [55] |
| *Fucus spiralis* | 9.71 | 5.23 | 17.59 | [63] |
| **Green seaweeds (Chlorophyceae)** | | | | |
| *Ulva compressa* | 15.7–32.1 | 1–1.7 | 14.5–79.9 | [58] |
| *Ulva lactuca* | 12–20 | 2–4 | 42–46 | [57] |
| *Caulerpa taxifolia* | 12.44 | 0.32 | 23.86 | [55] |

**Table 1.**
*Biochemical composition of seaweed families.*

Moreover, it has proven to be a sustainable alternative to traditional antibiotics, helping to prevent diseases and improve stress response [66]. Numerous research investigations have confirmed the function of microalgae as a feed additive [67], as they are a natural source of carotenoids, lipids, protein, and vitamins [68]. According to numerous reports, adding microalgae to the diet enhances intestine function, carcass quality, and several physiological activities while also increasing muscle protein, lipids, and omega-3 content [69]. Hassan et al. [70] reported that diets containing microalgae are a natural source of nutrients, contribute significantly to balanced nutrition, and are rich in essential proteins, omega-3 FAs, fats, vitamins, minerals, and antioxidants that positively affect growth and survival.

### *2.2.1 Biochemical composition of microalgae*

Microalgal have potential characteristics that make them an excellent ingredient acting as functional ingredients in aquafeeds; they have higher concentrations of EFAs such as EPA and DHA, high protein content, balanced AAs [71], and good sources of bioactive compounds, such as polyphenols and pigmentations [72]. The chemical composition of microalgae relies on various factors, such as the species and cultivation conditions; for example, *Arthrospira platensis* is high in protein content, whereas

| Microalgae species | Protein | Lipid | Carbohydrate | References |
|---|---|---|---|---|
| *Chlorella vulgaris* | 51–58 | 14–22 | 12–17 | [73] |
| *Chlorella pyrenoidosa* | 57 | 2 | 26 | [74] |
| *Acutodesmus obliquus* | 50–56 | 12–14 | 10–17 | [75] |
| *Arthrospira platensis* | 46–70 | 4–6 | 8–25 | [76–78] |
| *Arthrospira maxima* | 60–71 | 6–7 | 13–16 | [79] |
| *Phaeodactylum tricornutum* | 39.6 | 18.2 | 25.2 | [80] |
| *Dunaliella salina* | 49–57 | 6 | 32 | [81] |
| *Isochrysis galbana* | 27 | 36.6 | 34.5 | [82] |
| *Haematococcus pluvialis* | 48 | 14 | 24 | [83] |
| *Nannochloropsis oceanica* | 29 | 18–24 | 31–39 | [83] |

**Table 2.**
*Functional components (%) of different microalgae.*

Tisochrysis lutea is high in PUFA content [14, 72]. **Table 2** summarizes the biochemical composition of some microalgae species used in fish feed.

## 3. Growth and physiological response

**Tables 3, 4**, and **Figure 2** show the effects of algae on growth in fish and crustaceans.

### 3.1 Growth response and feed utilization

Modulating feed is crucial for enhancing fish growth, and the growth performance is controlled by a range of features, including water quality, temperature, diet chemical composition, types of ingredients, feed additives incorporated, and effective management practices [98]. Recently, several studies have shown that the inclusion of aquatic plants enhancement fish growth [99] in fish and crustaceans such as Nile tilapia [91], catfish [97], rainbow trout [87], Asian Seabass [51], hybrid red tilapia [13], and whiteleg shrimp [6, 19, 26]. Previous studies have concluded that the inclusion of algae in European sea bass [71], Nile tilapia [13], and whiteleg shrimp *L. vannamei* [19] enhance growth and feed utilization efficiency. Ashour et al. [6] revealed that including seaweed-based polysaccharides in shrimp diets resulted in enhancements in growth and growth-related gene expression versus basal diet. Follow the same patterns, Zeynali et al. [100] displayed that inclusion of seaweeds in aquafeeds enhanced growth and immunity response. The previous findings could be attributed to different scenarios such as (i) high content of bioactive compounds Manikandan et al. [100], (ii) algae act as an antioxidant compound [7], (iii) algae have plenty of polysaccharides that act as prebiotics that boost the growth of beneficial bacteria and banned the growth of harmful bacteria [26] and (iv) polysaccharides in algae act as growth promoters [24], and (v) the presence of sulfate carbohydrates in algae [13] that elevate immune system response and induce growth and feed efficiency [93]. On the contrary Silva-Breto et al. [101] and Shapawi and Zamry [102] reported that the inclusion of seaweeds had no significant effect on the growth of

| Seaweeds species | Aquatic animal species | Applied Levels | Effective Level | Period (Day) | Response | References |
|---|---|---|---|---|---|---|
| *Hypnea* sp. | Nile tilapia, *O. niloticus* | 0, 5, 10, 15, 20% | 10% | 90 | ↑Nutrient composition, ↑FA | [84] |
| *Sargassum dentifolium* | hybrid red tilapia | 0, 10, 20, 30 g/kg | 20 g | 84 | ↑FBW, ↑SGR, ↑FCR, ↑SR, ↑RBCs, ↑ Hb, ↑Hct, ↑Lipase, ↑↓ albumin, ↑creatinine, ↑GPT, ↑GOT, Cholesterol | [13] |
| *Dictyota dichotoma* | Zebrafish, *D. rerio* | 0, 0.25, 0.5, 1% | Up to 0.5% | 63 | ↑WBE, ↑WG, ↑SR, ↑ Ig, ↑ Lys, ↑SOD, ↑GST, ↑ SOD, ↑ immune-related genes, ↑ growth-related genes | [85] |
| *Ulva intestinalis* | Zebrafish, *D. rerio* | 0, 0.25, 0.5, 1% | 1% | 56 | ↑GPx, ↑SOD, ↑↓CAT, ↑growth-related genes | [86] |
| *Sargassum dentifolium* | Shrimp, *L. vannamei* | 0, 1, 2, 3 g/kg | 3 g/kg | 90 | ↑WG, ↑SR, ↑SOD, ↑GPx, ↑ProPO, ↑Lys↑growth-related genes, ↑ immune-related genes | [19] |
| *Galaxaura oblongata* | Rainbow trout, *O. mykiss* | 0, 0.5, 1% | 1% | 56 | ↑↓WG, ↑Ig, ↑ Lys, ↑CAT, ↑SOD, ↑GPx, ↑interleukin 6 (il-6), ↑ tumor necrosis factor- gene expressions | [87] |
| *G. pulvinata, S. ilicifolium* | Asian Seabass, *Lates calcarifer* | 0, 3, 6, 9, 12, 15% | 9–12% | 56 | ↑↓WG; ↑Lys, ↑SOD, ↑Liver igf-1, il-1β, il-8, ↑antioxidant status, ↑ FA | [51] |
| Mixer seaweed extract: *U, lactuca, P. capillacea, J. rubens* | Shrimp, *L. vannamei* | 0, 1, 2, 3, 4% | 2% | | ↑FW, ↑WG, ↑SGR, ↑FCR, ↑FER, ↑PER, ↑Lys, ↑SOD, ↑CAT, ↑ lipase, ↑amylase, ↑ immune-related genes | [6] |
| Mixer seaweed extract: *U, lactuca, P. apillacea, J. rubens* | Nile tilapia, *O. niloticus* | 0, 0.5, 1, 1.5, 2%, | up to 2% | 70 | ↑WG, ↑FU, ↑ ADG, ↑SGR, ↑SGR, ↑PI, ↑PER, ↑ PPV, ↑TP, ↑Lys, ↑ non-specific immunity | [23] |
| *Hypnea* sp | Nile tilapia, *O. niloticus* | 0, 5, 10, 15, 20% | 15% | 90 | ↑FW, ↑WG, ↑ immunity system, ↑ bactericidal activity | [52] |
| *Ulva* sp. | Nile tilapia, *O. niloticus* | 0, 10, 20, 30% | 10% | 60 | ↑FBW, ↑FI, ↑SGR, ↑FER, ↑SR, ↑protein retention, ↑ lipid retention, ↑erythrocytes, ↑leucocyte, ↑Hb, ↑Hct | [88] |
| *S. angustifolium* | Common carp, *Cyprinus carpio* | 0, 5, 10, 15 | 10–15 | 60 | ↑hepatic antioxidant enzymes, ↑ antioxidant-related genes, ↑ hepatic metabolic enzymes | [89] |
| *Ulva, Eisenia, Porphyra.* | Shrimp, *L. vannamei* | 0, 5, 10, 15% | Up15% | 28 | ↑ FBW, ↑FI, ↑digestive activity, ↑FU, ↑SR | [90] |

↑ : increase, ↓ : deficiency, ↑↓ : no effect. *FBW: final body weight (g), WG: weight gain (g), ADWG: average daily weight gain (g), FI: feed intake (g/kg), FU: feed utilization, SGR: Specific growth rate (%/day), FCR: Feed conversion ratio, FER: feed efficiency ratio, SR%: survival rate, TP: total protein, PI: protein intake, PER: protein efficiency ratio, PPV: protein productive value, FA: fatty acid, RBCs: red blood cell, WBCs: white blood cell, Hb: hemoglobin, Hct: hematocrits, GOT: Serum glutamic oxaloacetic transaminase, GPT: glutamic pyruvic transaminase, GST: glutathione S transferase, MDA: Malondialdehyde, GPX: glutathione peroxidase, SOD: superoxide dismutase, CAT: serum catalase, Ig: total immunoglobulin content, ProPO: Prophenoloxidase, Lys: Lysozyme.*

**Table 3.**
*Effects on characteristics of various cultured aquatic animals fed on seaweed enhanced diet.*

| Microalgae species | Aquatic animal species | Applied Levels | Effective Level | Period (Day) | Response | References |
|---|---|---|---|---|---|---|
| *Golenkinia longispicula* | Nile tilapia, *O. niloticus* | 0, 5, 10, 15 g/kg | 15 | 90 | ↑FBW, ↑SGR, ↑FCR, ↑SGR, ↑hematocrit, ↑Hb, ↑RBCs, ↑GPX, ↑SOD, ↑CAT, ↑Hct, ↑immune-genes expression | [91] |
| *Schizochytrium* sp. | Shrimp, *L. vannamei* | 25, 50, 75% | 75 | 84 | ↑growth performance, ↑carcass proximate | [92] |
| *Amphora coffeaeformis* | Nile tilapia, *O. niloticus* | 0,2,4,6% | 4 | 84 | ↑growth, ↑protein, albumin, ↑ triglycerides, ↑creatinine, ↑globulin, ↑ ↓cholesterol, ↑ ↓glucose, | [93] |
| *Cyclotella meneghenian*a | Nile tilapia, *O. niloticus* | 0,5,10,15 g/kg | Up to 10% | 60 | FBW, ↑SGR, ↑FCR, ↑PER, ↑Hb; ↑Htc, ↑SR, ↓triglyceride | [7] |
| *A. platensis* | Zigzag Eel, *M. armatus* | 0, 5, 10, 15, 20% | Up to 10% | 70 | ↑FBW, ↑lysozyme, ↑intestinal metabolism, ↑MDA, ↓SOD, ↑ metabolomics, ↑ antioxidant enzyme | [94] |
| *A. platensis* | Catfish, *Ompok pabda* | 0, 10, 15, 20, 25% | 15 | 56 | ↑FW, ↑WG, ↑SGR, ↑FI, ↑FCR, ↑PER, ↑SR, ↑EAA, ↑ NEAA | [95] |
| *N. oculata* | Nile tilapia, *O. niloticus* | 0, 3, 5, 8% | 8 | 184 | ↑ FU, ↑SGR, ↑FI, ↑FCR, ↑SR%, ↓feed cost | [96] |
| *A. platensis* | Catfish, *H. fossilis* | 0, 1, 3, 5% | 5% | 60 | ↑FBW, ↑WG, ↑ADWG, ↑PER, ↑FCR, ↑SGR, ↑RBCs; ↑SR, ↑WBCs, ↑hemoglobin, ↑disease resistance, ↑lymphocytes, ↑monocytes | [97] |

↑ : increase, ↓ : deficiency, ↑ ↓ : no effect. *FBW: final body weight (g), WG: weight gain (g), ADWG: average daily weight gain (g), FI: feed intake (g/kg), FU: feed utilization, SGR: Specific growth rate (%/day), FCR: Feed conversion ratio, FER: feed efficiency ratio, SR%: survival rate, TP: total protein, PI: protein intake, PER: protein efficiency ratio, PPV: protein productive value, FA: fatty acid, RBCs: red blood cell, WBCs: white blood cell, Hb: hemoglobin, Hct: hematocrits, GOT: Serum glutamic oxaloacetic transaminase, GPT: glutamic pyruvic transaminase, GST: glutathione S transferase, MDA: Malondialdehyde, GPX: glutathione peroxidase, SOD: superoxide dismutase, CAT: serum catalase, Ig: total immunoglobulin content, ProPO: Prophenoloxidase, Lys: Lysozyme, EAA: essential amino acids, NEAA: nonessential amino acids.*

**Table 4.**
*Effects on characteristics of various cultured aquatic animals fed on microalgae enhanced diet.*

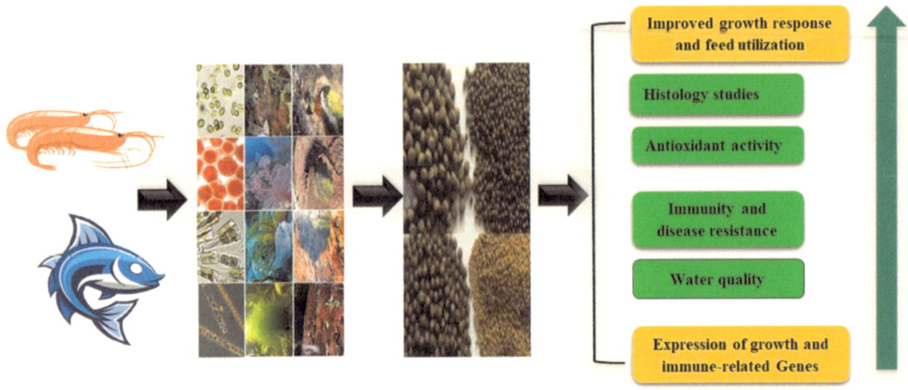
Improved growth response and feed utilization
Histology studies
Antioxidant activity
Immunity and disease resistance
Water quality
Expression of growth and immune-related Genes

**Figure 2.**
*Potential effects of algae utilization in aquaculture.*

seabream and Asian seabass. These contradictory results may be due to fish species, experimental conditions, seaweed species, and the doze of seaweed.

### 3.2 Body composition

One of the most important criteria for the retailer and consumer is the carcass chemical composition of fish [103]. Several factors affect the body's chemical nutrient composition such as seasons, gender, species and age [104]. Kumar et al. [105] showed that the inclusion of microalgae in shrimp diets had a significant impact on carcass chemical composition, resulting in high CP content and lower water and ash levels versus a basal diet formulation. Likewise, Ashour et al. [6] and Abbas et al. [19] revealed that inclusion of seaweeds in shrimp diets tended to increase CP content versus basal diet-fed fish. Since fish meal is expensive, less expensive but still appropriate substitutes are considered. Ringø [106] reported that, in finfish aquaculture, *Spirulina* may be a useful substitute supply of vitamins and protein. Moreover, Sultana et al. [107] and Taslima et al. [103] reported that the use of seaweeds and microalgae *Spirulina* improved the whole-body composition of Nile tilapia by increasing protein content. The present results could be attributed to two reasons, (i) high protein content of *Spirulina* and (ii) the ability of *Spirulina* to activate protein biosynthesis. Similar results were observed in *Trichopodus trichopterus* [108] and rainbow trout [109]. Recently, many research revealed that the inclusion of algae tended to increase body fat and FAs content, which has a vital role in preserving the body structure of different fish species [104]. Moreover, aquatic plants have been shown to have lipogenic enzyme activity and influence lipid metabolism in fish, including whole-body fat deposition and partitioning patterns [71]. Some studies have shown that algae have a high percentage of saturated and mono-saturated FAs, EPA and DHA [51, 71, 104].

### 3.3 Histology studies

Seaweeds can modify the gut microbial composition in animals and fish [110], by improving the villi structure and reducing the gut lumen of fish indicating a better ability to digest and assimilate feed nutrients by fish [65]. According to Sun et al. [94] and Abdelrhman et al. [13] these authors reported that enrichment the diets with microalgae enhances intestinal structure and function. Rahman et al. [97] revealed that the gut health of Nile tilapia was significantly improved in terms of structural integrity by incorporating different levels of *Spirulina* in the diet. Abdel-Moez et al. [7] reported that fish fed a diet supplemented with up to 10% *Spirulina* showed changes in goblet cell density, microvilli height, intraepithelial lymphocytes, and absorptive surface area. Similarly, compared to the control group, the length of the intestinal fold was significantly increased when 1–3% *Undaria pinnatifida* was added to shrimp *Penaeus monodon* diets [111]. These findings revealed that the algae diet had a positive impact on gut health [112].

### 3.4 Antioxidant activity

Fish health and antioxidant enzyme activity are tightly associated, and it becomes a crucial indicator of responses to oxidative stress [94]. To prevent oxidative damage to fish and crustacean tissues, which are typically affected by feed composition, this aspect needs to be fully addressed concerning advanced feed formulations. [26]. Oxidative stress has many adverse health effects and occurs when fish are exposed to unfavorable environments such as pollutants, viruses, and unfavorable temperatures [6]. The most significant antioxidant components reported in living organisms that are biomarkers for oxidative stress are a suite of specific enzymes, namely SOD, GST, and CAT [113]. The functions of these antioxidant enzymes vary. Superoxide ions are converted to hydrogen peroxide by SOD, while hydrogen peroxide breakdown and detoxification are facilitated by CAT and GPx. On the other hand, by the biochemical attaching of GSH to the xenobiotic, GST allows the xenobiotic detoxification process to occur [113]. Research on fish and crustaceans has demonstrated that diet compositions have a major impact on the activity of antioxidant enzymes. For example, algae contain potent bioactive compounds that have beneficial properties, such as antioxidant, anti-inflammatory, and immunomodulatory effects [65], they also can activate a wide range of enzymes, and contain an array of carotenoids, certain polysaccharides, and polyphenols that have scavenging activity against free radicals in tissues. According to recent research, algae can have a direct effect on the antioxidant status of fish by increasing antioxidant compounds or by enhancing the efficiency of primary cellular antioxidant defense systems.

Peixoto et al. [114], reported that adding 2.5% of the seaweed *Gracilaria* to the diet of European bass significantly enhanced glutathione peroxidase (GPx) activity [36]. Similarly, Abdelhamid et al. [13] displayed that hepatic oxidative enzyme activities were significantly higher in the seaweed-fed fish groups versus the basal diet. Moreover, Rouhani et al. [86] observed that zebrafish diets enriched with green macroalgae enhanced SOD and GPx activities. Furthermore, Liu et al. [50] noticed that the inclusion of algae (1 g/kg) promoted the activities of antioxidant enzymes of shrimp. Similarly, Kumar et al. [115] stated that the inclusion of algal meal in the shrimp diet boosted the enzymatic antioxidant capacity. The scenario behind the positive effect of algae on antioxidant enzyme activity could be attributed to the presence of bioactive compounds in algae that have antioxidant properties [13], and immunomodulatory, by strengthening the body's defense system and [36]. However, further researches are wanted to examine the aptitude of algae to protect fish from oxidative stress.

### 3.5 Immunity and disease resistance

Fish are highly susceptible and open to pathogen infection and diseases within intensive culture systems due to their interaction with their aqueous environment.

Consequently, this can cause negative impacts on health status and growth performance. Diseases are one of the main factors impeding the aquaculture industry's viability and profits, making disease resistance assessment critical. Therefore, strengthening the immune system of fish is crucial to controlling disease outbreaks [116]. However, the application of antibiotics has negative impacts on the aquaculture industry as the presence of resistant bacteria (AMR, antimicrobial resistance) will suppress the ability to control diseases due to the ineffectiveness of antibiotics used in aquaculture [36]. Therefore, research to find environmentally friendly components is needed in therapeutic strategies in fish farm husbandry. Recently, many research studies have highlighted the possibility of using algae and their bioactive compounds as a promising prophylactic and therapeutic substitute for conventional antibiotics [16, 93]. These are largely due to their positive properties as antiviral [117] antibacterial [86] and antioxidants [118], and consequently can raise and promote the immune system response [36]. For instance, the serum biochemical parameters are good markers to examine the capability of the immune system to protect from pathogen infection and control disease outbreaks [119]. Serum biochemical defense and stress indicators are some of the parameters that are considered crucial factors in promoting and boosting the immune system and blood functions in fish. They also serve as useful instruments for evaluating and monitoring nutritional-immune status [7, 15, 16, 93, 97].

Recent investigations have demonstrated that including algae in diet formulations of fish positively modulated fish immunity the defense mechanism, which helps fish increase their resistance to diseases, by increased Hb, Hct, RBC, WBC, and phagocytes. These results agree with [16] in *O. niloticus* [94], Zigzag Eel *Mastacembelus armatus* [120], red tilapia [13], and shrimp *L. vannamei* [6, 24]. Seyedalhosseini et al. [51] observed that serum immune parameters in fish fed with up to 9% of seaweed *Gracilaria* and *Sargassum* mixture were higher than in other treatments. Likewise, Mabrouk et al. [93] and Saleh et al. [121] revealed that inclusion of microalgae *A. coffeaeformis* in the diets of Nile tilapia fingerlings led to significant improvements in RBC, WBC, superoxide dismutase, catalase, aspartate transaminase, alanine transaminase, total serum protein, lymphocytes, monocytes, eosinophils, and lysozyme. Mendonca et al. [122] Mendonca et al. [107] reported that the use of 5% dietary *Gracilaria domingensis* algae improves the immune response of juvenile mullet. Mahmoudi et al. [52] showed that adding large red algae to the diet increased total immunoglobulin levels in fish. Ashour et al. [23] reported that adding different levels of seaweed as a dietary supplement enhanced the levels of TP, AL, and globulin in grey mullet and Nile tilapia, respectively. Seaweeds and microalgae are natural immunostimulants that increase fish immunity levels, by improving pathogen killing and resistance to infectious diseases in fish and shellfish [94, 123]. They will in the future become an important part in terms of advancing diets toward mitigation of diseases by offering a more comprehensive approach for building resilience through natural mechanisms [124, 125]. These functional novel ingredients can all play a vital role in supporting the welfare and sustainability agenda in aquaculture [45, 126].

### 3.6 Expression of growth and immune-related genes

Changes in fish metabolism, gene expression levels, and potential physiological effects following feed composition changes are explained by gene transcriptomics and metabolomics [94, 120]. Moreover, immune-related genes promote the production of inflammatory cytokines as well as cellular responses, causing the degradation of complex proteins [91]. Furthermore, GH and IGF-1 interact to control growth.

These are pleiotropic hormones that play a vital function in performance [127]. These gene expressions are controlled by different parameters like nutrition, environment as well as physiological and metabolic status [128]. Determining how environmental and nutritional factors influence the expression of GH and IGF-1 genes has great potential for improving fish health because the fish growth rate is a reflection of aquaculture productivity and profitability and associated dietary composition [86, 128], GH and IGF-1 have been used as an indicator of performance in aquaculture [86]. Seyedalhosseini et al. [51] reported that the relative expression level of igf-1 was higher in Asian seabream (*Lates calcarifer*) fed a diet containing 9% seaweed, which thereby indicates a physiological mechanism for better FER and growth performance. Similarly, Mahmoudi et al. [52] showed that zebrafish fed a macroalgae-rich diet showed significant dose-dependent upregulation of GH and IGF-1 genes. Liu et al. [129] and Rouhani et al. [86] noticed that shrimp and zebrafish-fed diets supplemented with seaweed upregulated both growth and immune-related gene expression respectively. Lee et al. [130] reported that the inclusion of a 5 g $kg^{-1}$ extract of *S. horneri* can induce upregulation of key innate immune gene expressions of *L. vannamei*. Similarly, Abbas et al. [19] reported that the incorporation level of S. dentifolium of 3 g/kg-1 enhanced immunity and stress-related gene expression in *L. vannamei*. Choi et al. [131] observed that dietary *Hizikia fusiformis* administration significantly increased plasma IGF-1 levels, which was accompanied by an increase in liver pro-inflammatory cytokines (IL-2 and IL-6) in juvenile olive flounder. Ashour et al. [24] and Abbas et al. [19] showed shrimp-fed diets supplemented with seaweed polysaccharide extract enhance the expression of growth, stress, and immune-related gene expression. These can all lead to improved performance of shrimp under intensive production and result in economic advantages.

### 3.7 Water quality

Water quality is a crucial factor that controls a number of characteristics of both a shrimp and a fish's nutrient assimilation and physiological state, with water degradation leading to aquaculture failure and the spread of diseases [65]. More recent research has confirmed the beneficial role of algae in aquaculture water treatment [132] through the process of biological treatment, efficient absorption of nutrients [133], conversion of highly toxic compounds into less biologically toxic chemicals, production of a variety of high-value compounds [115], oxygen generation, and regulation of the microbial community in water by absorbing pollutants and organic matter, further improving water quality, which leads to the promotion of biorefining processes for circular bioeconomy and sustainability in aquaculture practices [134]. According to Rahman et al. [97], the use of algae in aquaculture has been demonstrated to enhance water quality by absorbing nutrients such as phosphate and nitrogen, successfully reducing excess nutrient burdens, avoiding overfeeding, and reducing environmental damage. Depending on variables such as microalgae species, wastewater load, and additional $CO_2$, studies show that microalgae may remove a variety of pollutants from aquaculture wastewater, leading to much fewer hazards and toxicity events [129, 133].

## 4. Conclusion and future prospective

Compared to other alternatives, algae is a valuable marine resource that is used in a variety of ways as a replacement for fish oil and fishmeal. Moreover, due to its excellent nutritional profile, it has much potential for use as a feed ingredient in aquaculture. It is rich in many nutrients and functional bioactive compounds that are essential for fish growth and immunity. It also helps fish grow more effectively and strengthens their immune systems. Despite the potential advantages of algae, their economic viability is limited by their high cost and small scale of manufacture. Moreover, anti-nutritional factors contained in algae can form complexes with algae proteins, which greatly reduces the solubility of proteins, thus inhibiting their digestion and absorption, and high ash and moisture content leads to decreased digestibility of feed. Finally, as the production of algae worldwide is predicted to continue growing, so will the applications, demand, and elements of sustainable production. Therefore, there is also a need to invest in biotechnology for more efficient algae production systems and increase the availability of high-quality algae biomass, and more research to identify the most suitable algae species, optimum dose in aquafeeds, and also whether their inclusion is most appropriate when used as a secondary ingredient or functional additive.

## Acknowledgements

The open access of this work was supported by the UiT at the Arctic University of Norway, Norway.

## Conflict of interest

The authors declare no conflict of interest.

## Author details

Einar Ringø[1*], Mohamed Ashour[2], Sherine Ahmed[3], Zaki Sharawy[2], Ashraf Goda[2] and Ehab El-Haroun[3]

1 Faculty of Biosciences, Fisheries, and Economics, Norwegian College of Fishery Science, UiT The Arctic University of Norway, Tromsø, Norway

2 National Institute of Oceanography and Fisheries (NIOF), Cairo, Egypt

3 Fish Nutrition Research Laboratory, Faculty of Agriculture, Animal Production Department, Cairo University, Cairo, Egypt

*Address all correspondence to: einar.ringo@uit.no

## References

[1] Abbas EM, Ali FS, Desouky MG, Ashour M, El-Shafei A, Maaty MM, et al. Novel comprehensive molecular and ecological study introducing coastal mud shrimp (*Solenocera crassicornis*) recorded at the Gulf of suez, Egypt. Journal of Marine Science and Engineering. 2020;**9**:9

[2] Naylor RL, Hardy RW, Buschmann AH, Bush SR, Cao L, Klinger DH, et al. A 20-year retrospective review of global aquaculture. Nature. 2021;**591**:551-563

[3] da Mota JB, Neves TA, da Costa DP, Starling MC, de Amorim CC, Miranda-Filho KC. Emerging contaminants related to Brazilian aquaculture. Reviews in Aquaculture. 2025;**17**(1):e12967

[4] Magouz FI, Essa MA, Matter M, Mansour AT, Gaber A, Ashour M. Effect of different salinity levels on population dynamics and growth of the cyclopoid copepod *Oithona nana*. Diversity. 2021; **13**:190

[5] Magouz FI, Essa MA, Matter M, Tageldein Mansour A, Alkafafy M, Ashour M. Population dynamics, fecundity and fatty acid composition of *Oithona nana* (Cyclopoida, Copepoda), fed on different diets. Animals. 2021;**11**: 1188

[6] Ashour M, Al-Souti AS, Mabrouk MM, Naiel MA, Younis EM, Abdelwarith AA, et al. A commercial seaweed extract increases growth performance, immune responses, and related gene expressions in white leg shrimp (*Litopenaeus vannamei*). Aquaculture Reports. 2024;**36**:102154

[7] Abdel-Moez AM, Ali MM, El-gandy G, Mohammady EY, Jarmołowicz S, El-Haroun E, et al. Effect of including dried microalgae *Cyclotella menegheniana* on the reproductive performance, lipid metabolism profile and immune response of Nile tilapia brood stock and offspring. Aquaculture Reports. 2024;**36**: 102099

[8] Mansour AT, Ashry OA, Ashour M, Alsaqufi AS, Ramadan KM, Sharawy ZZ. The optimization of dietary protein level and carbon sources on biofloc nutritive values, bacterial abundance, and growth performances of whiteleg shrimp (*Litopenaeus vannamei*) juveniles. Life. 2022;**12**:888

[9] Rifna E, Rajauria G, Dwivedi M, Tiwari BK. Circular economy approaches for the production of high-value polysaccharides from microalgal biomass grown on industrial fish processing wastewater: A review. International Journal of Biological Macromolecules. 2024;**254**:126887

[10] Abo-Taleb HA, El-Feky MM, Azab AM, Mabrouk MM, Elokaby MA, Ashour M, et al. Growth performance, feed utilization, gut integrity, and economic revenue of grey mullet, *Mugil cephalus*, fed an increasing level of dried zooplankton biomass meal as fishmeal substitutions. Fishes. 2021;**6**:38

[11] Hoseinifar SH, Ashouri G, Marisaldi L, Candelma M, Basili D, Zimbelli A, et al. Reducing the use of antibiotics in European aquaculture with vaccines, functional feed additives and optimization of the gut microbiota. Journal of Marine Science and Engineering. 2024;**12**:204

[12] McKuin B, Kapuscinski AR, Sarker PK, Cheek N, Lim J, Sabarsky M. Comparative life cycle assessment of marine microalgae, *Nannochloropsis* sp. and fishmeal for sustainable protein ingredients in aquaculture feeds.

Elementa: Science of the Anthropocene. 2023;**11**:00083

[13] Abdelrhman AM, Ashour M, Al-Zahaby MA, Sharawy ZZ, Nazmi H, Zaki MA, et al. Effect of polysaccharides derived from brown macroalgae *Sargassum dentifolium* on growth performance, serum biochemical, digestive histology and enzyme activity of hybrid red tilapia. Aquaculture Reports. 2022;**25**:101212

[14] Elshobary M, Ashour M. Algae for aquaculture, recent technological applications. In: Value-Added Products from Algae, Phycochemical Production and Applications. Cham: Springer; 2023. pp. 525-561. DOI: 10.1007/978-3-031-42026-9_16

[15] Mabrouk MM, Ashour M, Labena A, Zaki MA, Abdelhamid AF, Gewaily MS, et al. Nanoparticles of *Arthrospira platensis* improves growth, antioxidative and immunological responses of Nile tilapia (*Oreochromis niloticus*) and its resistance to *Aeromonas hydrophila*. Aquaculture Research. 2022;**53**:125-135

[16] Mabrouk MM, Ashour M, Younis EM, AWA A-W, Bauomi MA, Toutou MM, et al. Arthrospira platensis nanoparticles dietary supplementation improves growth performance, steroid hormone balance, and reproductive productivity of Nile tilapia (*Oreochromis niloticus*) broodstock. PLoS One. 2024; **19**:e0299480

[17] Li W, Li X, Song C, Gao G. Carbon removal, sequestration and release by mariculture in an important aquaculture area, China. Science of the Total Environment. 2024;**927**:172272

[18] Vázquez-Romero B, Villar-Navarro E, Perales JA, Garrido-Pérez C, Ruiz J. Techno-economic analysis of using microalgae to treat streams from fish RAS farming and replace fish meal: A case study. Journal of Water Process Engineering. 2024;**59**:104904

[19] Abbas EM, Al-Souti AS, Sharawy ZZ, El-Haroun E, Ashour M. Impact of dietary administration of seaweed polysaccharide on growth, microbial abundance, and growth and immune-related genes expression of the Pacific whiteleg shrimp (*Litopenaeus vannamei*). Life. 2023;**13**:344

[20] Ashour M, Hassan SM, Elshobary ME, Ammar GA, Gaber A, Alsanie WF, et al. Impact of commercial seaweed liquid extract (TAM®) biostimulant and its bioactive molecules on growth and antioxidant activities of hot pepper (*Capsicum annuum*). Plants. 2021;**10**:1045

[21] Ashour M, Khairy HM, Bakr A, Matter M, Alprol AE. Seaweed liquid extract AS novel sustainable solutions for phycobioremediation plant germination, and feed additive for marine invertebrate copepod. Scientific Reports. 2024;**14**:29553

[22] Ashour M, Mabrouk MM, Abo-Taleb HA, Sharawy Z, Ayoub HF, Van Doan H, et al. A liquid seaweed extract (TAM®) improves aqueous rearing environment, diversity of zooplankton community, whilst enhancing growth and immune response of Nile tilapia, *Oreochromis niloticus*, challenged by *Aeromonas hydrophila*. Aquaculture. 2021;**543**: 736915

[23] Ashour M, Mabrouk MM, Ayoub HF, El-Feky MM, Zaki SZ, Hoseinifar SH, et al. Effect of dietary seaweed extract supplementation on growth, feed utilization, hematological indices, and non-specific immunity of Nile Tilapia, *Oreochromis niloticus* challenged with *Aeromonas hydrophila*.

Journal of Applied Phycology. 2020;**32**: 3467-3479

[24] Ashour M, Mabrouk MM, Mansour AI, Abdelhamid AF, Kader MFA, Elokaby MA, et al. Impact of dietary administration of *Arthrospira platensis* free-lipid biomass on growth performance, body composition, redox status, immune responses, and some related genes of Pacific whiteleg shrimp, *Litopenaeus vannamei*. PloS one. 2024;**19**: e0300748

[25] Mansour AT, Ashour M, Abbas EM, Alsaqufi AS, Kelany MS, El-Sawy MA, et al. Growth performance, immune-related and antioxidant genes expression, and gut bacterial abundance of Pacific white leg shrimp, *Litopenaeus vannamei*, dietary supplemented with natural astaxanthin. Frontiers in Physiology. 2022;**13**:874172

[26] Sharawy ZZ, Ashour M, Labena A, Alsaqufi AS, Mansour AT, Abbas EM. Effects of dietary *Arthrospira platensis* nanoparticles on growth performance, feed utilization, and growth-related gene expression of Pacific white shrimp, *Litopenaeus vannamei*. Aquaculture. 2022;**551**:737905

[27] Hosseini F, Hemmati A, Takabi FS, Naeini F, Bidar SS. A dose–response meta-analysis of randomized clinical trials investigating the effects of omega-3 supplementation on body weight in patients with cancer cachexia. Clinical Nutrition ESPEN. 2024;**59**:378-386

[28] Ashour M, Omran AM. Recent advances in marine microalgae production: Highlighting human health products from microalgae in view of the coronavirus pandemic (COVID-19). Fermentation. 2022;**8**:466

[29] Alprol AE, Mansour AT, Ibrahim MEED, Ashour M. Artificial intelligence technologies revolutionizing wastewater treatment: Current trends and future prospective. Water. 2024;**16**: 314

[30] Al-Saeedi SI, Ashour M, Alprol AE. Adsorption of toxic dye using red seaweeds from synthetic aqueous solution and its application to industrial wastewater effluents. Frontiers in Marine Science. 2023;**10**:1202362

[31] Ashour M, Alprol AE, Heneash AM, Saleh H, Abualnaja KM, Alhashmialameer D, et al. Ammonia bioremediation from aquaculture wastewater effluents using arthrospira platensis niof17/003: Impact of biodiesel residue and potential of ammonia-loaded biomass as rotifer feed. Materials. 2021; **14**:5460

[32] Ashour M, Alprol AE, Khedawy M, Abualnaja KM, Mansour AT. Equilibrium and kinetic modeling of crystal violet dye adsorption by a marine diatom, *Skeletonema costatum*. Materials. 2022;**15**:6375

[33] Ashour M, Mansour AT, Abdelwahab AM, Alprol AE. Metal oxide nanoparticles' green synthesis by plants: Prospects in phyto-and bioremediation and photocatalytic degradation of organic pollutants. PRO. 2023;**11**:3356

[34] Osman KM, Pires ÁDS, Franco OL, Orabi A, Hanafy MH, Marzouk E, et al. Enterotoxigenicity and antibiotic resistance of coagulase-negative *Staphylococci* isolated from raw buffalo and cow milk. Microbial Drug Resistance. 2020;**26**:520-530

[35] Madkour M, Matter IA, Abdelhady ARY, Alaqaly AM, Abd El-Azeem NA, Elsharkawy MS. Use of macro-and microalgae in animal nutrition. Organic Feed Additives for Livestock. 2025:107-125

[36] Siddik MA, Francis DS, Islam SM, Salini MJ, Fotedar R. Fermentation and fortification of *Sargassum linearifolium* with multi-strain probiotics improves mucosal barrier status, inflammatory response and resistance to *Vibrio harveyi* infection in barramundi *Lates calcarifer*. Aquaculture. 2025;**595**:741502

[37] Vijayaram S, Ringø E, Ghafarifarsani H, Hoseinifar SH, Ahani S, Chou C-C. Use of algae in aquaculture: A review. Fishes. 2024;**9**:63

[38] Aumeerun S, Soulange-Govinden J, Driver MF, Ranga RA, Ravishankar GA, Hudaa N. Macroalgae and microalgae: novel sources of functional food and feed. In: Handbook of Algal Technologies and Phytochemicals. Taylor & Francis Group, CRC Press; 2019. pp. 207-219

[39] Suganya T, Varman M, Masjuki H, Renganathan S. Macroalgae and microalgae as a potential source for commercial applications along with biofuels production: A biorefinery approach. Renewable and Sustainable Energy Reviews. 2016;**55**:909-941

[40] Griffiths M, Harrison ST, Smit M, Maharajh D. Major commercial products from micro-and macroalgae. Algae Biotechnology: Products and Processes. 2016:269-300. DOI: 10.1007/978-3-319-12334-9_14

[41] Kim SW, Shen G, Jacobsen C, Naseri A, Holdt SL, Loftus SE, et al. Seaweed and Microalgae as Alternative Sources of Protein. Vol. 107. Sawston, England: Burleigh Dodds Science Publishing; 2021

[42] Ashour M, Mansour AT, Alkhamis YA, Elshobary M. Usage of *Chlorella* and diverse microalgae for $CO_2$ capture-towards a bioenergy revolution. Frontiers in Bioengineering and Biotechnology. 2024;**12**:1387519

[43] Eladl SN, Elnabawy AM, Eltanahy EG. Recent biotechnological applications of value-added bioactive compounds from microalgae and seaweeds. Botanical Studies. 2024;**65**:28

[44] Chénais B. Algae and microalgae and their bioactive molecules for human health. Molecules. 2021;**26**:1185

[45] Ghosh S, Sarkar T, Pati S, Kari ZA, Edinur HA, Chakraborty R. Novel bioactive compounds from marine sources as a tool for functional food development. Frontiers in Marine Science. 2022;**9**:832957

[46] Menaa F, Wijesinghe U, Thiripuranathar G, Althobaiti NA, Albalawi AE, Khan BA, et al. Marine algae-derived bioactive compounds: A new wave of nanodrugs? Marine Drugs. 2021;**19**:484

[47] Cheong K-L, Yu B, Chen J, Zhong S. A comprehensive review of the cardioprotective effect of marine algae polysaccharide on the gut microbiota. Food. 2022;**11**:3550

[48] Alvanou MV, Loukovitis D, Melfou K, Giantsis IA. Utility of dairy microbiome as a tool for authentication and traceability. Open Life Sciences. 2024;**19**:20220983

[49] Martínez-Antequera FP, Martos-Sitcha JA, Reyna JM, Moyano FJ. Evaluation of the inclusion of the green seaweed *Ulva ohnoi* as an ingredient in feeds for gilthead sea bream (*Sparus aurata*) and European sea bass (*Dicentrarchus labrax*). Animals. 2021;**11**: 1684

[50] Yang S, Liu H, Guo W, Wang C, Sun C, Chan S, et al. Effects of salinity

and temperature on the metabolic and immune parameters of the banana shrimp *Fenneropenaeus merguiensis* (De Man, 1988). Iranian Journal of Fisheries Sciences. 2020;**19**:2010-2023

[51] Seyedalhosseini SH, Salati AP, Torfi Mozanzadeh M, Parrish CC, Shahriari A, Ahangarzadeh M. Effect of dietary seaweed (*Gracilaria pulvinata* and *Sargassum ilicifolium*) on serum and mucosal immunity, some growth and immune-related genes expression, antioxidant status, and fatty acid profile in asian seabass (*Lates calcarifer*). Aquaculture Nutrition. 2024;**2024**: 3683163

[52] Mohammad M, Sultana N, Begum A, Naser MN. Seaweed (*Hypnea* sp.) supplementation in feed play role in boosting immunity of Nile Tilapia (*Oreochromis Niloticus*). Dhaka University. Journal of Biological Sciences. 2022;**31**:177-181

[53] Masoomi-Feshani H, Vazirzadeh A. Long-term effects of probiotics on health biochemical indices of serum and mucus in rainbow trout (*Oncorhynchus mykiss*). Marine Reports (MAREP). 2022;**1**:1-12

[54] Olsson J, Toth GB, Albers E. Biochemical composition of red, green and brown seaweeds on the Swedish west coast. Journal of Applied Phycology. 2020;**32**:3305-3317

[55] Hentati F, Tounsi L, Djomdi D, Pierre G, Delattre C, Ursu AV, et al. Bioactive polysaccharides from seaweeds. Molecules. 2020;**25**:3152

[56] Marinho-Soriano E, Fonseca P, Carneiro M, Moreira W. Seasonal variation in the chemical composition of two tropical seaweeds. Bioresource Technology. 2006;**97**:2402-2406

[57] Mansour AT, Ashour M, Alprol AE, Alsaqufi AS. Aquatic plants and aquatic animals in the context of sustainability: Cultivation techniques, integration, and blue revolution. Sustainability. 2022;**14**: 3257

[58] Xie C, Lee ZJ, Ye S, Barrow CJ, Dunshea FR, Suleria HA. A review on seaweeds and seaweed-derived polysaccharides: Nutrition, chemistry, bioactivities, and applications. Food Reviews International. 2024;**40**: 1312-1347

[59] Fayaz M, Namitha K, Murthy KC, Swamy MM, Sarada R, Khanam S, et al. Chemical composition, iron bioavailability, and antioxidant activity of *Kappaphycus alvarezzi* (Doty). Journal of Agricultural and Food Chemistry. 2005;**53**:792-797

[60] Mandalka A, Cavalcanti MILG, Harb TB, Toyota Fujii M, Eisner P, Schweiggert-Weisz U, et al. Nutritional composition of beach-cast marine algae from the Brazilian coast: Added value for algal biomass considered as waste. Food. 2022;**11**:1201

[61] Samarasinghe M, Van Der Heide M, Weisbjerg M, Sehested J, Sloth JJ, Bruhn A, et al. A descriptive chemical analysis of seaweeds, *Ulva* sp., *Saccharina latissima* and *Ascophyllum nodosum* harvested from Danish and Icelandic waters. Animal Feed Science and Technology. 2021;**278**:115005

[62] Skrzypczyk VM, Hermon KM, Norambuena F, Turchini GM, Keast R, Bellgrove A. Is Australian seaweed worth eating? Nutritional and sensorial properties of wild-harvested Australian versus commercially available seaweeds. Journal of Applied Phycology. 2019;**31**: 709-724

[63] Paiva L, Lima E, Neto AI, Baptista J. Seasonal variability of the biochemical composition and antioxidant properties

of *Fucus spiralis* at two Azorean Islands. Marine Drugs. 2018;**16**:248

[64] Yang L, Yang Q, Hu R-G, Cong W, Li S, Kang Y-H. The evaluation of bacteriophage therapy in aquaculture: A systematic review and meta-analysis. Aquaculture. 2024:740925

[65] Rahman MT, Khan MA, Islam I, Dey MM. Trade credits in farming: A drain for gain in the aquaculture industry of Bangladesh. Aquaculture Economics & Management. 2023:628-642. DOI: 10.1080/13657305.2023.2289936

[66] Katsoulis-Dimitriou S, Nikouli E, Gkalogianni EZ, Karapanagiotidis IT, Kormas KA. The effect of dietary fish oil replacement by microalgae on the gilthead sea bream midgut bacterial microbiota. bioRxiv. 2024;**4**:e113

[67] Torres-Maravilla E, Parra M, Maisey K, Vargas RA, Cabezas-Cruz A, Gonzalez A, et al. Importance of probiotics in fish aquaculture: Towards the identification and design of novel probiotics. Microorganisms. 2024;**12**:626

[68] Sales R, Galafat A, Vizcaíno A, Sáez M, Martínez T, Cerón-García M, et al. Effects of dietary use of two lipid extracts from the microalga *Nannochloropsis gaditana* (Lubián, 1982) alone and in combination on growth and muscle composition in juvenile gilthead seabream, *Sparus aurata*. Algal Research. 2021;**53**:102162

[69] Flores-Moreno S, Vizcaíno A, Sáez M, Macías-Vidal J, Martínez T, Martos-Sitcha J, et al. Effects of phytase and microalgae supplementation on the utilization of aquafeeds for European seabass (*Dicentrarchus labrax*) formulated with a high inclusion level of plant protein. Aquaculture Research. 2024;**2024**:4775004

[70] Hassan MSA, Elias NA, Hassan M, Mocktar NA, Harun NA. Integrated overview on status, diagnosis and disease management of acute hepatopancreatic necrosis disease (AHPND) in shrimp aquaculture through metallic nanoparticles (MNPs) application–A review. Aquaculture. 2024:741649

[71] Mota CS, Pinto O, Sá T, Ferreira M, Delerue-Matos C, Cabrita AR, et al. A commercial blend of macroalgae and microalgae promotes digestibility, growth performance, and muscle nutritional value of European seabass (*Dicentrarchus labrax* L.) juveniles. Frontiers in Nutrition. 2023;**10**:1165343

[72] Jadhav HB. Functional triacylglycerols from microalgae and their use in the formulation of functional foods–Review. Food Chemistry Advances. 2024;**4**:100695

[73] Viegas C, Gouveia L, Gonçalves M. Evaluation of microalgae as bioremediation agent for poultry effluent and biostimulant for germination. Environmental Technology & Innovation. 2021;**24**:102048

[74] Prajapati SK, Malik A, Vijay VK. Comparative evaluation of biomass production and bioenergy generation potential of *Chlorella* spp. through anaerobic digestion. Applied Energy. 2014;**114**:790-797

[75] Ansari F, Ratha S, Renuka N, Ramanna L, Gupta S, Rawat I, et al. Effect of microplastics on growth and biochemical composition of microalga *Acutodesmus obliquus*. Algal Research. 2021;**56**:102296

[76] Gao K, Ma Z. Photosynthesis and growth of *Arthrospira* (*Spirulina*) *platensis* (Cyanophyta) in response to

solar UV radiation, with special reference to its minor variant. Environmental and Experimental Botany. 2008;**63**:123-129

[77] Barkia I, Saari N, Manning SR. Microalgae for high-value products towards human health and nutrition. Marine Drugs. 2019;**17**:304

[78] Borowitzka MA. Microalgae in medicine and human health: A historical perspective. In: Microalgae in Health and Disease Prevention. Elsevier, ScienceDirect; 2018. pp. 195-210

[79] Becker EW. Microalgae for human and animal nutrition. In: Handbook of Microalgal Culture: Applied Phycology and Biotechnology. Hoboken, New Jersey: John Wiley & Sons; 2013. pp. 461-503

[80] Tibbetts SM, Milley JE, Lall SP. Chemical composition and nutritional properties of freshwater and marine microalgal biomass cultured in photobioreactors. Journal of Applied Phycology. 2015;**27**:1109-1119

[81] Chen Y, Tang X, Kapoore RV, Xu C, Vaidyanathan S. Influence of nutrient status on the accumulation of biomass and lipid in *Nannochloropsis salina* and *Dunaliella salina*. Energy Conversion and Management. 2015;**106**:61-72

[82] He Y, Lin G, Rao X, Chen L, Jian H, Wang M, et al. Microalga Isochrysis galbana in feed for *Trachinotus ovatus*: Effect on growth performance and fatty acid composition of fish fillet and liver. Aquaculture International. 2018;**26**: 1261-1280

[83] Siddiqui SA, Ucak İ, Afreen M, Sasidharan A, Yunusa BM, Bhowmik S, et al. Microalgae as a potential raw material for plant-based seafood alternatives: A comprehensive review. Food Science & Nutrition. 2024

[84] Sultana Z. Histological alterations in the kidney of Nile tilapia (*Oreochromis niloticus*), exposed to Celecron 50EC. Journal of Agriculture, Food and Environment (JAFE). 2024;**5**:30-34, ISSN (Online Version): 2708-5694

[85] Mahmoudi N, Safari R, Shabani A, Hoseinifar SH, Yazici M, El-Haroun E. Can dietary *Dictyota dichotoma* powder affect performance, serum, and mucus immune parameters, and antioxidant defense in Zebrafish (*Danio rerio*)? Aquaculture Reports. 2022;**26**:101279

[86] Rouhani E, Safari R, Imanpour MR, Hoseinifar SH, Yazici M, El-Haroun E. Effect of dietary administration of green macroalgae (*Ulva intestinalis*) on mucosal and systemic immune parameters, antioxidant defence, and related gene expression in zebrafish (*Danio rerio*). Aquaculture Nutrition. 2022;**2022**:7693468

[87] Yazici M, Zavvar F, Hoseinifar SH, Nedaei S, Doan HV. Administration of red macroalgae (*Galaxaura oblongata*) in the diet of the rainbow trout (*Oncorhynchus mykiss*) improved immunity and hepatic gene expression. Fishes. 2024;**9**:48

[88] Suryaningrum LH, Samsudin R. Nutrient digestibility of green seaweed Ulva meal and the influence on growth performance of Nile tilapia (*Oreochromis niloticus*). Emirates Journal of Food and Agriculture. 2020;**32**:488-494

[89] Brontowiyono W, Jasim SA, Mahmoud MZ, Thangavelu L, Izzat SE, Yasin G, et al. Dietary (macro-algae, *Sargassaceae*) extract improved antioxidant defense system in diazionon - exposed common carp. Annals of Animal Science. 2022;**22**:1323-1331

[90] Omont A, Elizondo-González R, Escobedo-Fregoso C, Tovar-Ramírez D, Hinojosa-Baltazar P, Peña-Rodríguez A. Bacterial communities and digestive enzymatic activities of *Litopenaeus vannamei* shrimp fed pre-digested seaweeds as a functional ingredient. Journal of Applied Phycology. 2021;**33**: 1239-1251

[91] Moawad DA, El-Garhy HA, Refaat MH, Hassaan MS. Protecting deleterious effects of high stocking density of Nile tilapia, *Oreochromis niloticus* using dietary microalgae *Golenkinia longispicula*: Growth, immune-oxidative markers and associated gene expression. Aquaculture. 2024;**581**:740430

[92] Kumar V, Habte-Tsion HM, Allen KM, Bowman BA, Thompson KR, El-Haroun E, et al. Replacement of fish oil with *Schizochytrium* meal and its impacts on the growth and lipid metabolism of Pacific white shrimp (*Litopenaeus vannamei*). Aquaculture Nutrition. 2018;**24**:1769-1781

[93] Mabrouk M, Ashour M, Abdelghany MF, Elokaby MA, Abdel-Warith AWA, Younis EM, et al. Effects of dietary supplementation with benthic diatom *Amphora coffeaeformis* on blood biochemistry, steroid hormone levels and seed production efficiency of Nile tilapia *Oreochromis niloticus* broodstock. Journal of Animal Physiology and Animal Nutrition. 2024;**108**(6):1605-1615

[94] Sun D, Wang C, Wu H, Wang D, Xiang W, Zou J. Effects of replacing fishmeal with *Spirulina platensis* powder on the Zig-zag eel (*Mastacembelus armatus*): Growth performance, flesh quality, digestibility, and gut microbial composition. Aquaculture Reports. 2024; **37**:102263

[95] Akter T, Hossain A, Rabiul Islam M, Hossain MA, Das M, Rahman MM, et al. Effects of Spirulina (*Arthrospira platensis*) as a fishmeal replacer in practical diets on growth performance, proximate composition, and amino acids profile of pabda catfish (*Ompok pabda*). Journal of Applied Aquaculture. 2023;**35**: 69-82

[96] Sarker PK, Kapuscinski AR, McKuin B, Fitzgerald DS, Nash HM, Greenwood C. Microalgae-blend tilapia feed eliminates fishmeal and fish oil, improves growth, and is cost viable. Scientific Reports. 2020;**10**:19328

[97] Rahman M, Al Mamun MA, Rathore SS, Nandi SK, Kari ZA, Wei LS, et al. Effects of dietary supplementation of natural *Spirulina* on growth performance, hemato-biochemical indices, gut health, and disease resistance to Aeromonas hydrophila of Stinging catfish (*Heteropneustes fossilis*) fingerling. Aquaculture Reports. 2023; **32**:101727

[98] Ragab M, El-Diasty M, El-Sherbini M, AbdelKhalek A. Effect of *Spirulina* on somatic cell count and milk quality. Journal of Advanced Veterinary Research. 2023;**13**:637-642

[99] Serra DR, Floh EI, Chow F. Metabolic changes of the red marine alga *Gracilariopsis tenuifrons* elicited by high PAR in laboratory. Brazilian Journal of Botany. 2024;**47**:585-596

[100] Zeynali M, Nafisi Bahabadi M, Morshedi V, Ghasemi A, Torfi Mozanzadeh M. Replacement of dietary fishmeal with *Sargassum ilicifolium* meal on growth, innate immunity and immune gene mRNA transcript abundance in *Lates calcarifer* juveniles. Aquaculture Nutrition. 2020;**26**: 1657-1668

[101] Silva-Brito F, Guardiola FA, Cavalheri T, Pereira R, Abreu H,

Kijjoa A, et al. Dietary supplementation with *Gracilaria* sp. by-products modulates stress response, antioxidant and immune systems of gilthead seabream (*Sparus aurata*) exposed to crowding. Journal of Applied Phycology. 2020;**32**:4347-4359

[102] Shapawi R, Zamry AA. Response of Asian seabass, *Lates calcarifer* juvenile fed with different seaweed-based diets. Journal of Applied Animal Research. 2016;**44**:121-125

[103] Taslima K, Selly SLC, Mc Andrew BJ, Penman DJ. Combined estrogen and elevated temperature treatments induce feminization in Nile tilapia, *Oreochromis niloticus*. Aquaculture Reports. 2023;**33**:101773

[104] Sultan MB, Rahman MM, Khatun MA, Shahjalal M, Akbor MA, Siddique MAB, et al. Microplastics in different fish and shellfish species in the mangrove estuary of Bangladesh and evaluation of human exposure. Science of the Total Environment. 2023;**858**: 159754

[105] Kumar VE, Ravikumar G, Jeyasanta KI. Occurrence of microplastics in fishes from two landing sites in Tuticorin, South east coast of India. Marine Pollution Bulletin. 2018; **135**:889-894

[106] Ringø, E, Spirulina platensis, A Functional Feed Additive in Finfish Aquaculture–An Update; 2024.

[107] Sultana N, Mohammad M, Lisa SA, Saha B, Begum M, Naser MN. Effects of dietary inclusion of Seaweed in regular commercial fish feed on proximate composition, minerals and fatty acid profiling of Nile Tilapia Oreochromis niloticus (Linnaeus, 1758). Aquatic Food Studies. 2022;**2**(2):AFS112. DOI: 10.4194/AFS112

[108] Khanzadeh M, Esmaeili Fereidouni A, Seifi Berenjestanaki S. Effects of partial replacement of fish meal with *Spirulina platensis* meal in practical diets on growth, survival, body composition, and reproductive performance of three-spot gourami (*Trichopodus trichopterus*) (Pallas, 1770). Aquaculture International. 2016;**24**: 69-84

[109] Teimouri M, Yeganeh S, Amirkolaie A. The effects of *Spirulina platensis* meal on proximate composition, fatty acid profile and lipid peroxidation of rainbow trout (*Oncorhynchus mykiss*) muscle. Aquaculture Nutrition. 2016;**22**: 559-566

[110] Cerezo IM, Fumanal M, Tapia-Paniagua ST, Bautista R, Anguís V, Fernández-Díaz C, et al. *Solea senegalensis* bacterial intestinal microbiota is affected by low dietary inclusion of *Ulva ohnoi*. Frontiers in Microbiology. 2022;**12**: 801744

[111] Niu J, Chen X, Lu X, Jiang S-G, Lin H-Z, Liu Y-J, et al. Effects of different levels of dietary wakame (*Undaria pinnatifida*) on growth, immunity and intestinal structure of juvenile *Penaeus monodon*. Aquaculture. 2015;**435**:78-85

[112] Ferreira M, Ogren M, Dias JN, Silva M, Gil S, Tavares L, et al. Liposomes as antibiotic delivery systems: A promising nanotechnological strategy against antimicrobial resistance. Molecules. 2021;**26**:2047

[113] Yousefsaber F, Hosseini Abari A, Bahrami A, Abbasi MS. Improving the Bioactivity, Biocompatibility, and Antimicrobial Properties of Bioactive Glass Coating with the Addition of Pectic Oligosaccharide, Obtained from Microbial Degradation. Available at SSRN: https://ssrn.com/abstract= 4972509. DOI: 10.2139/ssrn.4972509

[114] Peixoto MJ, Magnoni L, Gonçalves JF, Twijnstra RH, Kijjoa A, Pereira R, et al. Effects of dietary supplementation of *Gracilaria* sp. extracts on fillet quality, oxidative stress, and immune responses in European seabass (*Dicentrarchus labrax*). Journal of Applied Phycology. 2019;**31**: 761-770

[115] Kumar VS, Pandey P, Anand T, Bhuvaneswari GR, Dhinakaran A, Kumar S. Biofloc improves water, effluent quality and growth parameters of *Penaeus vannamei* in an intensive culture system. Journal of Environmental Management. 2018;**215**:206-215

[116] Maldonado-Miranda JJ, Castillo-Pérez LJ, Ponce-Hernández A, Carranza-Álvarez C. Summary of economic losses due to bacterial pathogens in aquaculture industry. In: Bacterial Fish Diseases. Elsevier; 2022. pp. 399-417

[117] Klongklaew N, Praiboon J, Tamtin M, Srisapoome P. Chemical composition of a hot water crude extract (HWCE) from *Ulva intestinalis* and its potential effects on growth performance, immune responses, and resistance to white spot syndrome virus and yellowhead virus in Pacific white shrimp (*Litopenaeus vannamei*). Fish & Shellfish Immunology. 2021;**112**:8-22

[118] Harikrishnan S, Parivallal M, Alsalhi MS, Sudarshan S, Jayaraman N, Devanesan S, et al. Characterization of active lead molecules from *Lissocarinus orbicularis* with potential antimicrobial resistance inhibition properties. Journal of Infection and Public Health. 2021;**14**: 1903-1910

[119] Fazio F. Fish hematology analysis as an important tool of aquaculture: A review. Aquaculture. 2019;**500**:237-242

[120] Sun D, Hou D, Zheng Y, Xiang W, Huang Y, Wu H, et al. Multi-omics reveals the effects of spirulina platensis powder replacement of fish meal on intestinal metabolism and stress in zig-zag eel (*Mastacembelus armatus*). Antioxidants. 2024;**13**:851

[121] Saleh NE, Ismail RF, Sayed AEDH, Zaghloul EH, Saleh H. Comprehensive assessment of benthic diatom (*Amphora coffeaeformis*) as a feed additive in Nile tilapia (*Oreochromis niloticus*) diet. Aquaculture Research. 2020;**51**: 3506-3519

[122] Mendonça AJC, Rosas VT, Monserrat JM, Romano LA, Tesser MB. The inclusion of algae *Gracilaria domingensis* in the diet of mullet juveniles (*Mugil liza*) improves the immune response. Journal of Applied Aquaculture. 2019;**31**:210-223

[123] Mohammadiazarm H, Zehirikia Y, Kalantarzadeh S, Etehadi K, Salati AP, Mousavi SM, et al. Growth, body composition, digestive enzyme activity, blood biochemical parameters, and immune antioxidant indices of red tilapia fish (*Oreochromis mossambicus* × *Oreochromis niloticus*) reared in mixed cell and rectangular raceways. Aquaculture Reports. 2023;**33**:101803

[124] Olabi A, Shehata N, Sayed ET, Rodriguez C, Anyanwu RC, Russell C, et al. Role of microalgae in achieving sustainable development goals and circular economy. Science of the Total Environment. 2023;**854**:158689

[125] Cai J, Lovatelli A, Aguilar-Manjarrez J, Cornish L, Dabbadie L, Desrochers A, et al. Seaweeds and microalgae: an overview for unlocking their potential in global aquaculture development. FAO Fisheries and Aquaculture Circular. 2021

[126] Ndebele-Murisa MR, Mubaya CP, Dekesa CH, Samundengo A, Kapute F, Yossa R. Sustainability of aqua-feeds in Africa. Sustainability. 2024;**16**:10323

[127] Caputo M, Pigni S, Agosti E, Daffara T, Ferrero A, Filigheddu N, et al. Regulation of GH and GH signaling by nutrients. Cells. 2021;**10**:1376

[128] Triantaphyllopoulos KA, Cartas D, Miliou H. Factors influencing GH and IGF-I gene expression on growth in teleost fish: how can aquaculture industry benefit? Reviews in aquaculture. 2020;**12**:1637-1662

[129] Liu W-C, Zhou S-H, Balasubramanian B, Zeng F-Y, Sun C-B, Pang H-Y. Dietary seaweed (*Enteromorpha*) polysaccharides improves growth performance involved in regulation of immune responses, intestinal morphology and microbial community in banana shrimp *Fenneropenaeus merguiensis*. Fish & Shellfish Immunology. 2020;**104**:202-212

[130] Lee M-K, Ryu H, Lee JY, Jeong HH, Baek J, Van JY, et al. Potential beneficial effects of *Sargassum* spp. in skin aging. Marine Drugs. 2022;**20**:540

[131] Choi YH, Kim K-W, Han H-S, Nam TJ, Lee B-J. Dietary *Hizikia fusiformis* glycoprotein-induced IGF-I and IGFBP-3 associated to somatic growth, polyunsaturated fatty acid metabolism, and immunity in juvenile olive flounder *Paralichthys olivaceus*. Comparative Biochemistry and Physiology Part A: Molecular & Integrative Physiology. 2014;**167**:1-6

[132] Han Q, Zhao S, Zhang X, Wang X, Song C, Wang S. Distribution, combined pollution and risk assessment of antibiotics in typical marine aquaculture farms surrounding the yellow sea, North China. Environment International. 2020;**138**:105551

[133] Ling T-Y, Tan A-C, Nyanti L, Sim S-F, Grinang J, Ganyai T. Seasonal variations in water quality of a tropical reservoir: considerations for cage aquaculture expansion. Aquaculture, Aquarium, Conservation & Legislation. 2018;**11**:333-347

[134] Hashemi SS, Abbasi-Riyakhuni M, Denayer JF, Tabatabaei M, Aghbashlo M, Karimi K. Efficient bioremediation of distillery and dairy wastewaters: A three-stage biorefinery for high-quality aquaculture feed and bioenergy generation. Process Safety and Environmental Protection. 2023;**180**:566-574